the
7-MINUTE MIRACLE

the 7-MINUTE MIRACLE

THE BREAKTHROUGH
PROGRAM TO
BANISH SPOT FAT
FOREVER

Sheldon Levine, M.D.

LifeLine
Press
A Regnery Publishing
Company
Washington, D.C.

Library of Congress Cataloging-in-Publication Data on file

First paperback printing 2003

ISBN 0-89526-182-0

Published in the United States by
LifeLine Press
A Regnery Publishing Company
One Massachusetts Avenue, NW
Washington, DC 20001

Visit us at www.lifelinepress.com

Distributed to the trade by
National Book Network
4720-A Boston Way
Lanham, MD 20706

Printed on acid-free paper
Manufactured in the United States of America

10 9 8 7 6 5 4 3 2 1

Books are available in quantity for promotional or premium use. Write to Director of Special Sales, Regnery Publishing, Inc., One Massachusetts Avenue, NW, Washington, DC 20001, for information on discounts and terms or call (202) 216-0600.

To Sarah Merewald and Helen Kurland
Two aunts who left me their magical legacy.

CONTENTS

Introduction/xv

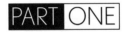

PART THREE

WHAT ARE YOU DOING THE REST OF YOUR LIFE?

ACKNOWLEDGMENTS

I thank Janette, Alison, and David, who make today even more special than yesterday. I can't wait until tomorrow.

My parents, Bella and Sol Levine, continue their solid, unwavering support, as Dr. Ilana Rindner nurtures us with her wisdom, as does the spirit of Richard Rindner.

And Arlene and Uri Ascher and Marc Rindner Esq., I admire you all.

My agent always gets top billing after the family. Mel Berger, thanks.

None of us would be here now without the terrific folks at LifeLine Press, beginning with Mike Ward, Associate Publisher, who got this project jumping, then saw it through with his vision right up to the end. Mike, thank you.

Editor Molly Mullen, drawing on her experience as a writer and marathoner, got people and paper together on time and in the "write" mix. Thanks, Molly.

Art director Rich Kershner designed *The 7-Minute Miracle* from cover to cover. His immense talent, like this book, are open for all to see. Thanks, Rich.

Publicist Lauren Lawson (another marathon runner!) gets the word out from East coast to West and beyond. Having her on your side gives an author a much-needed advantage in the book world. Good going, Lauren.

John Lalor of Special Sales and Marketing is imagination personified, creating spins where none existed before, while Shadi Akhavan, Marketing Associate, brought insight and energy to the project. I thank these two creative LifeLiners.

Jack Croft, freelance editor, is special. He drafted a light, airy quality to the manuscript, organizing it, making it easily accessible. Well done, Jack, even though you are in Philly accent denial!

Laurie Schlussel, R.D., M.A., is the brains behind the menus. A true professional, she worked within the tightest of deadlines and never complained. Thanks Laurie.

Lada St. Edmund, personal trainer extraordinaire, advised me on the workout routines in the book. Terrific, Lada. Heather Henry and Scott Grimaldi brought the routines to life with style. Thanks, guys.

Betty Del Pozzo and Judy D'Andrea guard my sanity in Mahwah and are cherished.

I will miss the lively conversations with the late John Cammarata, M.D., a bariatric pioneer, almost as much as his patients miss him. I thank his wife Kathy for her support.

Kudos to Elizabeth Letizia.

Spencer Delisle, Anne Dittamo, Detective Jack Oppelt, Mary Jo McFadden, Darlene Clark, Tracy Garrison, Stephanie Klein, Andrew Lesnak, Robbin Leibowitz, and Eric Mathews all helped in a big way. Thank you all.

Brad Adams and Donna Carrazone, former Mrs. New Jersey, deserve gratitude for their efforts.

Thanks to Claudia Allocco, Head Medical Librarian at the Valley Hospital, for help with the research for this book.

ACKNOWLEDGMENTS

A special salute to Sylvester Collins, Pvt. E-1, U.S.M.C., of Detroit. You'll find his name on Panel 13W, Line 73 on a low, black wall in Washington, D.C.

Thank you to Pam from Great Expectations Antiques.

Finally, to all of my patients. The word "doctor" is derived from the Latin word for teacher. All my patients must be doctors, then, because they have taught me so much. Thank you all!

INTRODUCTION

Hi!

Brief introductions rule, don't you agree?

If you have an oversized body part that you wish were smaller, your time has come.

The same couldn't be said just a few short years ago. New discoveries in the fields of genetics and weight loss give us amazing fresh insights into how we lose weight, compelling us to change the very way we look at our bodies and body fat.

The latest research reveals that if you want trimmer thighs, hips, arms, and backsides, you'll first have to get off the high-protein, high-fat, low-carb merry-go-round. If you want to shrink your belly or buttocks, put your dumbbells down and get off your home exerciser. Saddlebags, spare tires, thunder thighs, and love handles are not the result of poor diet or poor exercise habits.

They are genetic!

And like genetic traits, fat accumulates at the same exact spots within families. That's why the lament "I have my father's backside" or "My thighs and hips are shaped just like my aunt's" can be heard throughout the land.

Think of it like this, your face resembles that of a relative because of genes and so does your body.

But if you are unhappy about a particular body part, don't curse your heredity, work with it!

The *7-Minute Miracle* introduces you to genetic body sculpting, a combination of eating and exercising in a specific way that targets fat only, not muscle.

Most body-shaping plans put too much emphasis on weight-lifting and muscle-building and not nearly enough on fat-burning. The unique genetic approach of *The 7-Minute Miracle* does away with weights, gyms, exercise machines, and round-the-clock dieting.

Your weight-control genes are normally dormant. But the 7-Minute Miracle Genetic Body Sculpting Plan wakes them up! Once you learn how, in just minutes, you can activate and reprogram the weight control genes from your least favorite body part. That's how you lose weight *when* you want to and, for the first time, from *where* you want to.

And it won't take forever, either.

The true miracle is what your body can accomplish in only 7 minutes, sparking a chain reaction that lasers in on and burns fat for hours, in the exact area that bugs you most, be it the hips, thighs, belly, butt, or arms.

This isn't fantasy, it's science.

The same science that demonstrates that no matter what your weight loss track record is, you can have your own private 7-Minute Miracle.

Go for it!

Best Wishes,

Sheldon Levine, M.S., M.D.
April, 2002

PART ONE

THE
NEW SCIENCE
OF GENETIC
WEIGHT LOSS

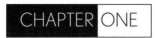

SCULPTING YOUR OWN MASTERPIECE IN 7 MINUTES A DAY

When the great Italian Renaissance artist Michelangelo set out to create his statue of David, he was careful not to re-create the super-muscular dudes with bulging pecs favored by the Greeks and Romans of antiquity.

Though he was only 29 years old, Michelangelo was 500 years ahead of his time in realizing that the stone physiques of yore were too stylized and unrealistic. He wanted the real deal, someone with a body that we all could relate to. So he hewed away tons of excess "fat," in the form of excess marble, to reveal the beauty of David's muscles beneath.

He may not have known it, but Michelangelo was also half a millennium ahead of his time in demonstrating a simple yet profound truth that—even today—is not understood by the self-proclaimed weight-loss gurus: That fat—not muscle—shapes you. If you want a shapely figure, you don't need lots of muscle. You need less fat.

Why? Because fat, not muscle, shapes the outer contours of your

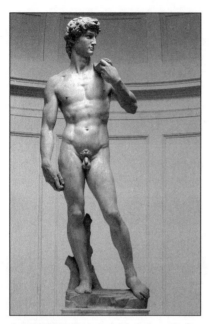

MASTERPIECE: It took Michelangelo 3 years to work a miracle with marble and reveal the flawless physique of "David."

body, determining how you look both in clothes and without them.

Consider this: The great block of Carrara marble that Michelangelo used to carve his colossal 13-foot David was not only a second-hand hunk of stone, it was actually a third-hand piece. Two other artists, Agostino di Duccio and Antonio Rossellino, had already worked on it before each eventually abandoned the project.

By decree of the town council, the marred marble was set outside in the courtyard of the Cathedral of Florence to face the elements for over 20 years! In 1501, the marble was rescued by Michelangelo, who took the old, flawed piece of stone, one with limited potential, trimmed it down, and—over the next 3 years—created a true rock of ages.

Your body has been through a lot and may be flawed, too. But like Michelangelo's stone, it has amazing potential. And you don't need a hammer and chisel to reveal the masterpiece within you. And you sure don't need three years.

All you need is 7 minutes a day.

21ST CENTURY WEIGHT LOSS

The 7-Minute Miracle is a scientifically based program that can help you sculpt your own masterpiece by chiseling away fat from the most troublesome areas of your body: your belly, hips, thighs, butt, and arms.

That fat is so important is based on a simple anatomical observation. What you see and feel first when you examine your body is fat. Body fat lies on top of muscle, right beneath your skin. Your muscles lie deeper, underneath the fat.

To have a chiseled and sculpted body, you need to remove the layer of accumulated fat that covers up your muscles. And that's what The 7-Minute Miracle does: Using the latest scientific discoveries about the key role that genetics plays in how much you weigh, it focuses your body's natural weight-loss abilities like a laser on one spot, the body part that troubles you most.

This is the face of 21st century weight loss.

The 7-Minute Miracle combines a precise exercise and eating plan to specifically target the fat you want to get rid of. Seven minutes of moving your body, followed by a great-tasting meal, revs you up to burn fat throughout the day, whether you are driving, reading, or sitting on the couch watching TV.

There are two things you *won't* do as part of The 7-Minute Miracle: You won't walk, and you won't lift weights. Both, quite frankly, are a waste of time as far as weight loss is concerned. I know that runs counter to what you've heard from almost every other supposed weight-loss expert, but I'll show why it's true.

Sounds like a miracle, doesn't it? But it's not. It's pure science.

So before we get to the program itself, let me explain how and why this program works. Because I don't want you to just take my word for it. After all, I'm from Brooklyn, so I know that when someone says, "Trust me," you should reach for your wallet to make sure it's still there. Lots of very smart people in white lab coats have devoted lots of time to studying how the body works to come up with this program.

As important as the scientific studies are, though, I don't want you to think this program has only been tested in the lab. I know it works because not only have I seen the scientific proof, I've seen the amazing results in people just like you—people who have chiseled away the fat to reveal the beautiful sculpture underneath.

THE APPLE AND THE GRAPEFRUIT

To understand why this fat-blasting program works, you first need to understand how fat and muscle work. Although fat and muscle are close neighbors, they are separate body tissues with little in common. They have separate metabolisms and even separate genes. Their differences begin with their biochemical makeup.

Skeletal muscle is organized into lengths of tightly knit, well-organized protein strands, called fibers, that contract and relax together on voluntary command. Fat, on the other hand, is made up of a loose confederation of fat-filled cells that move only when you wiggle or jiggle them, on purpose or not! The fat in fat cells has the consistency of expandable foam rubber. That's why fat is far less dense than muscle and occupies up to five times more space than muscle of equal weight.

To see the difference, let's turn to our national pastime—baseball. A pound of muscle is about the size of a hardball, while a pound of

The Weight Training Paradox

Suppose your thighs are too thick and flabby to suit you. No doubt, thigh muscle makes up some of the thickness, but let's be real here: It's not *all* muscle.

Your thighs stick out because globs of fat that sit on top of your thigh muscles force your skin to stretch and protrude outwardly. The thigh muscles beneath just go along for the ride.

In fact, those of you who have tried weight training to correct a similar thigh problem have probably been confronted by a definite biological paradox: Weight training builds an even thicker layer of thigh muscles, pushing against your layer of thigh fat, which makes your thighs protrude still further.

That's why I say that building more muscle is not the answer. Burning more fat is.

fat is roughly the size of a softball. Or, to use a comparison from the produce section of your local supermarket, a pound of muscle is about the size of a medium apple, while a pound of fat is the size of a medium grapefruit.

Now you can begin to understand how losing even a single pound of fat from a strategic area can change the entire way you look. Just imagine the difference if you could scoop a softball-sized chunk of fat off your belly, butt, thighs, hips, or arms. But don't just imagine it. Do it, with The 7-Minute Miracle Genetic Body Sculpting Plan, which includes a short but intense workout, a strategic break, and a delicious meal.

THE 7-MINUTE MIRACLE WORKOUT

To flatten your belly, trim your thighs, or slim your hips, you don't have to join a gym or lift a single weight. There's no need to build new muscle tissue, because you get great results with the muscles you already have.

In fact, with my 7-Minute Miracle Workout, you don't exercise to build muscle. You exercise to burn fat. And while you're burning fat, you boost your metabolism and sense of well-being, while actually decreasing your appetite. All of these benefits are yours if you give me just 7 minutes a day.

That's because deep inside you, on the microscopic level, your fat cells are all set to burn fat from your tough-luck spots. And it only takes 7 minutes' worth of special gene-activating exercises to get them going.

Actually, most of the fat you burn occurs *after* you exercise, not during it.

No matter what your level of physical fitness, flexibility, or dexterity, and no matter how much muscle you have, in only 7 minutes you can begin the process that will ultimately force your fat to hit the highway.

But let me say up front that these 7-minute workouts are no cakewalk. They are intense. If you do them right, you'll work up an honest sweat, guaranteed. Sweating body fluids, that's fine, but sweating your cash, isn't.

That's why you don't have to buy any of the wacky, house-clogging, space-hogging equipment as seen on TV. They remind me of steel scarecrows, scaring people away from using them. And few people do.

Besides, there are far better places to hang your wet laundry.

THE 7-MINUTE MIRACLE MEAL

My favorite diet joke goes like this:

> I once asked a patient what kind of diet she was on.
> "Oh, I'm on three diets now," she answered.
> "Why three?"
> "Because I don't get enough food on one diet!"

No one wants to diet, right?

So don't.

Can you imagine a future without dieting? You'd better start, because you don't diet to spot reduce. You *eat* to spot reduce. Instead of worrying about what you'll eat the whole day, it's much easier to concentrate on just one meal a day: The 7-Minute Miracle Meal.

It's based on the simple premise that *when* you eat counts as much as *what* you eat. The spot meal, eaten just once a day, consists of eating only those foods that energize your weight control genes, coaxing them into burning fat. But it only works if the meal follows the 7 minutes of specialized exercises. Because what you eat *before* exercise does not cause spot weight loss, but what you eat *after* exercise, does! At least it does if it's The 7-Minute Miracle Meal.

It doesn't matter whether you eat the target meal for breakfast, lunch, or dinner. Just so long as it's the meal you eat after exercising. And within reason, it doesn't matter what you eat the other two meals of the day. This intimate and essential link between gene-activating exercise and fat-busting foods makes up the genetic fat attack unique to The 7-Minute Miracle.

And as with most things in life, timing is everything. In this case, the timing of the meal is precisely 40 minutes after your workout. Once again, there's sound scientific reason for this strategic break.

It's only been in recent years that science has begun to understand how important a role genetics plays in weight loss. We now know that most people aren't overweight because they're weak or lack sufficient willpower. Their bodies are genetically programmed to gain weight in certain areas. So enough with the guilt trips. Even if you feel like you weren't blessed with the greatest genetics, don't curse your heredity. Work with it.

I'll show you how.

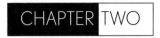

CHAPTER TWO

FACING
THE FACTS OF FAT

Before you can begin burning off unwanted fat, you first need to understand what it is and the important role it plays in your body.

Much as Jacques Cousteau's underwater explorations changed our view that oceans are just giant basins of liquid and fish, the electron microscope and gene technology provide us with a new look at fat and fat cells.

It's now clear that fat cells and the genes they contain control multiple body functions in a fashion that was undreamed of a few years ago. Your body has 30 billion fat cells, each containing about one-billionth of a pound of fat. That comes out to 30 pounds of body fat for the average, normal-weight person.

Overweight people have more fat in their cells, while the obese may have more total fat cells than those who aren't overweight.

Fat cells are as near and dear to your body as heart or kidney cells. They're just as important, too. They are very busy little factories, open 24/7, manufacturing leptin, interleukin 6, and properdin—substances that modulate your immune system, fight against infection and cancer, cause weight loss, and control fertility.

Keep in mind that your fat cells are not isolated. They work together and are in close contact with your brain, stomach, intestines, liver, pancreas, and sexual organs. Depending on their size, a hot spot like your thighs or belly can contain millions of fat cells.

It's also clear that all fat is not created equal. Fat at the hips, for instance, is different from fat around the abdomen. Fat around the upper back is different from fat around your arms. These differences may have profound health implications for you, as you'll soon see.

Fat even comes in different colors, like brown and white. And that's another crucial difference.

Brown fat is scarce in quantity, but high in quality. Found mostly around your body's major artery, the aorta, and between the shoulder blades, brown fat manufactures proteins that control metabolism.

One of these proteins, *uncoupling protein*, may hold promise as a powerful "exercise pill" to treat obesity, because it tricks your body into acting as if it's exercising even while you eat! It's being tested right now in the laboratory.

Most body fat is white.

There are two types of white fat: superficial fat, which makes up three-quarters of all body fat, and core fat. Core fat lies deeper, is tougher, and seems to literally stick to your ribs. It serves as the body's last-ditch depot against starvation, so it's closely guarded by intricate biochemical systems to maintain itself.

There is one special type of core fat that deserves a second look: visceral fat.

DON'T WAIST YOUR LIFE

In 1985, Swedish researcher P. Bjorntorp described the male "apple" and female "pear" body-fat distribution patterns. His research hinted

Fat Fit For a Priest

For thousands of years, we've craved the taste of fat. Don't take my word for it. It's in the Bible.

In Leviticus, the third book of the Old Testament, whole sections recount how the Israelite priests are entitled to their share of globs of sacrificial fat. For example, Leviticus chapter 7, verse 3, describes a typical ancient offering: "And he (the priest) shall offer of it, all the fat thereof; the fat tail, and the fat that covereth the inwards."

Fat gets mentioned three times in just one sentence! That's major billing!

Subsequent verses empower the priests to eat the burnt fat and meat, making the priests the first to ever try the Atkins Diet!

Hopefully, God took care of the priest's cholesterol!

at a connection between your belly fat and a deeper layer of fat that surrounds your intestines, called visceral fat.

This is *the* bad boy of fats. That's why it's nicknamed "heart-attack fat." Unlike other body fat, visceral fat contains some scary-sounding substances like tumor necrosis factor that contribute to high blood pressure, adult-onset diabetes, high cholesterol and, of course, heart attacks.

Using high-resolution CAT scans, researchers have corroborated that the more visceral fat you have, the greater your risk for serious cardiovascular disease. This is particularly true for adult-onset diabetes, which affects 16 million people in this country alone.

The diabetes epidemic is so out of hand that every sixty seconds, another person gets diagnosed with diabetes. There are actually seven million people walking around right now with diabetes who don't even know that they have it!

An estimated 90 percent of adult-onset diabetes cases are related to being overweight and to abdominal visceral fat in particular. So it's absolutely essential to know whether you have this fat time bomb ticking inside you.

How do you know if you have too much of this hidden fat? It's simple: If you have excess belly fat, there is good chance that you also have a proportional excess of the deeper fat. And that means a greater chance of serious health problems.

Lose your belly fat and you actually lower your risks!

With these relationships in mind, medical scientists came up with a healthy waist size for you. Like knowing your cholesterol or your spouse's birthday, it's a number that you must be aware of:

Men: Keep your waistline below 40 inches.

Women: Keep your waistline below 35 inches.

Who would have thought that losing as little as one inch off your waist could make you healthier!

That was a deep medical discussion. Let's get more superficial, because when it comes to weight loss, superficial fat is where it's at.

A FANTASTIC FAT VOYAGE

Spot fat, the stuff that gives you love handles and flabby arms, is 100 percent superficial fat. Let's take one cell out, miniaturize ourselves, and see what it looks like, up close and personal.

Each fat cell is round and has small projections sticking out of it like a balding porcupine. Inside the cell is one snowball of fat, called glycerol. This fatty snowball will melt and leave the fat cell to get burned up (as free fatty acids) if it's given the signal to do so by an enzyme also located in the fat cell, called *hormone-sensitive lipase*.

The process of releasing fat from the fat cells on top of your muscles is known as lipolysis, (pronounced li-POL-e-sis), which comes from the Greek for "fat breakdown." It's amazing when you think about it: Twenty-five hundred years ago, the Greeks recognized the profound differences between fat and muscle.

If lipolysis sounds vaguely familiar, it should: Liposuction, in the end, does the same thing, getting rid of excess fat. The big difference is that lipolysis is natural, without risk or pain, is cost-free, and can be done at home. Tough choice, huh?

I've said that lifting weights won't help you lose weight and get the body you want. This is one of the reasons: Lipolysis has *nothing* to do with building muscle, a process known as hypertrophy. Lipolysis is a catabolic, or breakdown, function of the body, while hypertrophy is a build-up, or anabolic, body function.

Lipolysis involves the breakdown of fat tissue only, leading to fat loss and increased muscular definition. Hypertrophy, on the other hand, in-

Hypertrophy vs. Lipolysis

Here is a quick chart to help clarify the main differences between muscle building (hypertrophy) and fat breakdown (lipolysis)

	MUSCLE BUILDING	FAT BREAKDOWN
Definition	Muscle growth	Fat release
Metabolic process	Anabolic (build-up)	Catabolic (breakdown)
Where it works	Muscle tissue	Fat cell
Action	Muscle development	Fat loss
Weightlifting	Bigger muscles	No direct effect
7-Minute Miracle Plan	Muscle definition	Shrink fat spots

As you can see, the column on the left is all about muscles and muscle-building, the column on the right is all about fat and fat loss. This reflects the fundamental fact that they are two separate processes. Though fat is ultimately burned in muscle tissue, no fat-burning can occur without fat breaking down and leaving the fat cell first.

As you can also see, unlike weightlifting—which only works to make your muscles bigger—The 7-Minute Miracle not only gets rid of excess fat, it defines your muscles at the same time.

volves muscle tissue only and leads to muscle growth, but no fat loss.

HITTING THE G-SPOT

Lipase, the enzyme in your fat cells that gives the all-clear sign for fat to make a break for it, is usually like a lazy lion snoozing on the savanna. Most of the time, it just hangs out. Until it gets activated.

Are you with me so far? Good.

The projections on the surface of the cell are like tiny fishing rods. They're called receptors, because, well, they receive things. These receptors have an on-off switch known as G-protein, also located outside the cell.

If you want to burn fat, the G-protein outside the fat cell must be turned on first. That sends a signal to the inside of the cell to activate the lipase, which sends fat packing.

Did you ever dream that this is what's going on in just one cell out of millions on your thighs, right now? Wow! This frenetic action, which you are totally oblivious to, is also occurring at the other hot spots on your body: your belly, butt, hips, and thighs.

Then who's watching the store?

Your genes are!

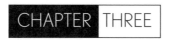
THE NEW SCIENCE OF GENETIC WEIGHT LOSS

You probably discovered weight-control genes before the scientists did.

Every time you looked in the mirror and said, "Wow, I have my mother's thighs," or "Yikes, I'm looking at my grandmother's tush," you were feeling the power of your genes.

It's all part of what I call "the genetic spot-fat continuum." Spot fat passes continuously like an invisible chain letter, from an ancestor of a previous generation to you. The letter is written in DNA, and the postman who delivers the letter is your genes.

Long ago, certain weight-control genes entered your family's bloodline. Today, these same genes help determine not only how much, but *where* your body stores fat. How you look in your jeans depends on the look of your genes!

And remember, these genes are ancient. They were already old when they went, two by two, on a free Mediterranean cruise, courtesy of Captain Noah. Your genes come not only from your parents, but from their great-great-great-grandparents and beyond. That means you may even have your Neanderthal aunt's thighs!

Another sign that genetics and weight are inextricably linked is that serious regional weight gain often follows definitive genetic milestones such as puberty, menopause, and, particularly, after childbirth. Each day in this country there are 10,000 births. One out of every four new moms will go on to weigh more after delivery than before she became pregnant. The post-partum period will be her defining moment on the road to overweight or obesity.

Incredibly, these new moms usually gain the same amount of weight that their mothers did and pack it on in the exact same places, like the hips and thighs!

Over the years, you may lose hundreds of pounds. Unfortunately, you also find them again. No doubt you've noticed that each time you regain weight, it is slapped on to the exact same site, in the same order, each and every time!

It was only in 1994 that science discovered why this happens. That year, Jeffrey M. Friedman, M.D., and his team at Rockefeller University in New York City, isolated the first weight-control gene, called the ob (short for "obesity") gene.

Dr. Friedman's research opened all of our eyes to a new view of weight control, which can be summed up in one sentence: Weight loss is regulated by genes, not willpower.

HOW YOUR GENES WORK

Remember those 30 *billion* fat cells your body has? Well, each one contains multiple weight-control genes. Genes are like loyal watchdogs, standing on guard to prevent fat from leaving your toughest areas. No fat leaves the fat cell without their say-so.

Your weight-control genes are tiny, double-stranded ribbons of nucleic acid located deep inside your fat cells. They determine how and where fat is deposited on your body.

If your gene pool has received the primordial directive to turn your

The 10 Pillars of Genetic Weight Loss

1. Random exercise does not cause spot weight loss.
2. Exercise combining and exercise sequencing does.
3. Too much exercise increases appetite.
4. The increase in appetite is for carbs and fat.
5. Seven minutes of intense exercise decreases appetite.
6. Walking does not cause weight loss.
7. What you eat after exercise can slim you down.
8. Eating the wrong foods after a workout puts weight on.
9. Most fat-burning occurs after, not during, exercise.
10. A 40-minute food pause after exercise boosts weight loss.

thighs and bellies into genetic fat strongholds, then that's what happens. If the same gene pool is present in other family members, the same thing will happen to them.

Against thousands of years of genetic programming, a few hours at the gym or the latest fad diet has no chance.

When Robin P., a 27-year-old computer programmer from the Bronx, tells me, "I can't do anything with my Russian weightlifter arms. I look like the Michelin Woman," she's feeling the frustration of fighting against her own genetics. And when Steven G., a 40-year-old mechanic, tells me he gave up going to the gym because no matter how many sit-ups he does, "My belly still looks pregnant," he's expressing his own exasperation with the genes he was dealt.

Trying to beat your genes is like trying to beat yourself, because genes aren't just a big part of you, they *are* you!

That's why you can't outsmart them, you can't outrun them, and you certainly won't outlast them. But your genes aren't mute like sphinxes and they aren't totally set in their ways. Genes are flexible and will adapt to changing body conditions brought about, for instance, by intense exercise and diet.

With The 7-Minute Miracle, you can reprogram your genes to help you lose fat, not add fat. In fact, that's the only way it *can* happen, because if your spot fat is deposited genetically, it must come off genetically.

The true miracle revealed by the new gene science is that your weight-control genes are interactive. They respond in real time to what you eat and how you move.

The old view of genes being stone immutable is just that, old. The new view is that our body functions have a genetic basis and that most genes react to changes in your body's internal environment.

When you lift weights, for example, your muscles grow because genes in your muscles promote the growth process. Smokers get lung and bladder cancer because carcinogens in cigarettes cause genes to mutate, causing abnormal cell growth.

Genes are influenced by diet, too. The Japanese have a very high incidence of stomach cancer. As a nation, they consume lots of smoked meats and fish, which are high in nitrosamines, carcinogens that cause genes in cells of the stomach lining to turn cancerous.

Whether a child grows to his or her full physical potential depends on nutrition, exercise, sleep, and overall health, all of which influence genes to either help or hinder growth.

So to recap: Genes are interactive. They influence you. You can influence them.

Rodney Dangerfield jokes that his body is in such bad shape that it can't be donated to science. His has to be donated to science fiction, instead!

To spot reduce, you don't have to be a gene science genius, nor must you clone yourself and start over again. Everything you need to lose your spot fat is contained, like a good TV dinner, inside, so that you can eat and exercise your extra fat away, all by yourself, naturally!

By combining just 7 minutes a day of gene-energizing exercises with specific gene-energizing foods, you can give that extra spot of fat on your belly, hips, thighs, arms, or butt the old heave-ho, even as you lose weight from other parts of your body, too.

AN OLD ERROR, A NEW ERA

I like to think of weight loss before the discovery of the gene as the Before Gene (BG) Era. The initials also could stand for the *Blame Game Era*, or, to be more precise, *Error*, because we blamed weight-loss failure on anything that moved: insulin, blood type, carbohydrate addiction, protein, food color, bad calories, even bad spouses.

We have now entered the After Gene (AG) Era. The vital role played by weight-control genes is now an established scientific fact. Since the original weight-loss gene discovery, more than three thousand weight-loss gene-related research articles have been published, all pointing to a dynamic, new view that weight loss is largely governed by genetics.

But for me, two pieces of research that appeared within months of each other stand out. They are the ones that got the spot reducing ball rolling.

First, came mind-blowing research from French researchers that proves that the types of food you eat can alter your own weight-loss genes and the internal makeup of your fat cells.

The French scientists discovered that genes can be activated by certain foods, while other foods put them to sleep, closing the door on spot weight-reducing. The 7-Minute Miracle Meal Plan, in Part Two, shows you exactly what to eat to activate your genes to release the fat on your thighs, hips, belly, butt, and arms.

Once it was established that certain foods activate your weight-control genes, the question posed was: "Does exercise have the same gene-altering effect as food?" Other pioneering scientists answered this question with a resounding yes.

This time, French and American scientists figured out that exercise stimulates weight-control genes to promote fat-burning and weight loss in a previously unknown way. Since this groundbreaking research first appeared, thousands of corroborating and expanding studies have been published demonstrating that what you eat and how you exercise can influence your genes.

So the question is, how do you trigger your genes to start dumping fat from your fat cells? What wakes up the sleeping lion of lipase? It's the spark that ignites the fat-burning cascade within your targeted body part. It's adrenaline, the official hormone of The 7-Minute Miracle Genetic Body Sculpting Plan. I'll fully discuss the important role that adrenaline plays when we get to the Genetic Body Sculpting Plan in Part Two.

But for now, this revolution in gene science reveals sweeping new weight-loss concepts that I want to share with you.

Soon, you will be working with your own genes and using these new concepts as part of The 7-Minute Miracle Genetic Body Sculpting Plan that lets you exercise and eat away the excess fat from your most troublesome body part.

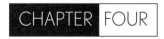

THE FIVE
HOT SPOTS FOR FAT

In the war against weight gain, spot fat is the enemy. And we don't need spies or high-tech surveillance equipment to discover where it hides. It's right there, in plain sight, on your body's five hot spots: your belly, butt, thighs, hips, and arms.

And here's the latest report from the scientific front: You don't control the five hot spots. Each is ruled by the weight-control genes inside your fat cells, which have enough power to turn those hot spots into five fat fortresses, fighting you tooth and nail to keep fat exactly where it is, diet or no diet, exercise or no exercise.

Your genes act like magnets that attract muscle-covering fat to the fat cells of each of the five hot spots, ultimately expanding your hips, thighs, belly, tush, and arms. What's more, your genes—not you—control what part of your body weight is lost from. The latest scientific breakthroughs have cracked the secret code that your genes use to signal how and where fat should be stored, and how and where it should be set free.

In a bizarre twist straight out of an *X-Files* episode, the secret code forms an ancient shape—the shape of a pyramid.

THE PYRAMID SCHEME

Here's what happens.

Once you get beyond your early twenties, your metabolism slows, signaling your body to store fat with vigor, progressing from the bottom up. Starting with your buttocks, hips, and thighs, your body's fat deposits creep upwards over your lifetime through the abdomen, arms, and eventually toward the narrow, upper part of your body—the face and neck.

If you think about it, the pattern of storing fat resembles a pyramid, with the wide base along your butt, thighs, and hips, going up to the top, your head. With less fat at the top parts of your body and more fat at the bottom and central abdominal areas, you get the classic "middle-age spread."

Each of you has your own individual weight-gain pyramid. While you may have more fat on your hips and thighs, your best friend may have more on her butt. But the basic pyramid framework holds true for everyone.

Your personal pyramid also depends on your sex. Men and women have different pyramids, thanks to different hormones at work. Female sexual hormones, like estrogen and progesterone, and male hormones, especially testosterone, influence where fat is stored. In general, men have more fat around the gut and women have more fat around their thighs and arms. The triceps area seems to be the hot spot most heavily influenced by the interaction of female hormones and genes.

It's a fact of life that women have more fat, percentage-wise, on their bodies than men. This discrepancy begins early in life, and by their mid-twenties, overweight women already outnumber overweight men two to one, a sex gap that increases with age. The difference between the sexes is based on the fact that women have larger breasts, which are mostly fat, and more rounded and fleshy backsides, shoulders, thighs, and hips.

Yet when it comes to losing spot fat, there *is* equality of the sexes, and both men and women have equal potential to lose their spot fat.

IT'S ONLY NATURAL

The location of your spot fat and your overall body shape are not random. They're as orderly as Charles Darwin's notebook. Nature tries hard to maintain the structural integrity of your pyramid by keeping fat safe and secure at each of the five hot spots.

You probably never thought about it quite like this, especially when you are forced to buy the next size larger jeans, but the five hot spots are part of a living, natural selection process that tries to protect you. The pyramid configuration offers an evolutionary advantage to those having fat on the bottom parts of their body, the base of the pyramid. Here's why:

Having extra weight (but not too much!) along your body's base lowers your center of gravity and adds stability and ballast, making locomotion (walking and running) easier.

There are other advantages, too. Fat on the lower part of your body shields vital organs, including parts of the large and small intestines, the spleen, and your sexual organs. It also acts like insulation, conserving body heat, especially in colder climates.

Recently it was discovered that fat on the lower body (again, not too much!) also fosters fertility and aids a developing fetus. In fact, many female world-class marathoners and triathletes who have too little fat on their lower body have lifelong problems with their menstrual cycles, and sometimes cannot conceive.

Another way to look at it is that the body can only devote so much

Debunking the Big-Boned Theory

Fat and muscle aren't the only things that shape your body contours. Bones have a big say in what your fat hot spots look like and, of course, in your overall body structure.

There are three basic body types, which I'll describe briefly:

MESOMORPHS: Those who are naturally thick and heavily muscled. Dr. Michael Anchors, author of *Safer Than Phen-fen!*, once told me that if you can't wrap your right hand around your left wrist, then you may be a meso-morph!

ECTOMORPHS: Those who are naturally thin and lanky.

ENDOMORPHS: Those with soft, round bodies like the Pillsbury Dough Boy. They generally lack muscle tone.

As you can see, there are profound differences in bone structure between the three groups. Whether you are a thick-boned mesomorph, or a thin-boned ectomorph, or an endomorph in-betweener, your bones are a scaffold responsible for your height and internal width. These physical parameters can't be changed with current technology. You can't make yourself taller or shorter, and you can't compress a wide pelvis or shoulder girdle.

What *can* be changed, no matter what your body type, are your body contours.

energy to fat storage. So it prioritizes and protects those areas that will increase the chances for survival in times of famine or starvation.

FIRST ON, LAST OFF

Perhaps the most ingenious thing about this pyramid scheme is how it reacts when you lose weight. The pyramid doesn't crumble, it automatically shifts into reverse. The rule for fat storage has bedeviled dieters for ages: First on, last off.

Have you noticed that when you lose weight, first your face gets

Whether you are short and stocky, tall and thin, or rounder than a quarter-pounder, you can slim down your hips if they jut out like two peninsulas. If your belly is making it difficult to see your shoes, spot weight loss can give you an unobstructed view once more.

Still, the bone structure issue comes up at least ten times a day in my practice. Overweight patients often look me straight in the eye and tell me that they are overweight because they are big-boned.

It reminds me of a story told by the comedian and actor Denis Leary:

A woman goes to her physician. "Doctor," she says, futilely attempting to circle her left wrist with her right hand. "As you can see, I'm heavy because I'm big-boned." The doctor looks at her wrists, smiles and answers, "Brontosauruses are big-boned, my dear. You are just heavy."

Many of my patients give more credence to the "big-boned theory" than the "big-bang theory." My take on the whole bone structure issue is this: You won't change your raptor-sized spot fat deposits until you change your dinosaur-like thinking about being bone-disadvantaged.

Save for the soft central marrow, bones are mostly solid columns of calcium. Once you have attained your full adult size, bone size cannot, in normal health, be altered.

But spot fat can. And that can make all the difference in how you look.

thinner, then—if you stick with the program long enough—weight loss gradually moves downward to the lower parts of your body? With a symmetry established eons before the last treasure was stolen from King Tut's tomb, fat loss begins at the top of the pyramid, your face and neck, and heads south. That's why it's so hard to lose the weight you most want to lose: around your belly, hips, butt, and thighs.

At some point in your diet or exercise plan, when your willpower fades or you hit a natural plateau, your weight loss slows and then stops. And the fat that stubbornly clings to hot spots like your thighs, tush, hips, and belly stands as fleshy sentinels, reminding us that we are victims of an ancient, genetic pyramid scheme.

OBESE OR NOT OBESE, THAT IS THE QUESTION

For an increasing number of Americans, the pyramid scheme doesn't stop at overweight. It keeps piling on the pounds until you cross the line into obesity. And that, my friends, can be scary territory.

In 1998, the National Institutes of Health estimated that 97 million Americans are overweight or obese. In reality, I almost never use the "O" word. It's all part of the rules of engagement in the weight-loss field, where it's taboo to throw the word obesity around freely.

Throughout my career, I can count on one hand the number of times that the word obese came up during a patient visit. Most obese people I've worked with are stuck in denial about themselves and their loved ones, particularly children and spouses. They see others as obese, but not themselves or their families, who—they tell me—may have just a "small weight problem."

So how do you know when you've crossed the line? If you look in the mirror and see lots of hot spots, unless they're measles or hives, you may have more than a just a local body fat problem. Ditto if you have a positive "pinch test" (see page 46) at more than three hot spots.

You might then be one of the many patients who ask, "Dr. Levine, what am I? Am I…you know, am I, like…overweight? I can't be obese because my brother-in-law is obese and he has a belly from here to Chicago. I don't."

Obese or not obese? Everyone with a weight problem wants to know. What patients really want is not so much an answer, but confirmation of a deep fear: that they are obese.

"Deep down, I know I'm not obese," you may be saying to yourself. "But I want the official word from the medical community. Do I get the big 'O' stamp for obesity, the little 'o' for overweight, or the 'N' for normal weight?"

The only known practical way to determine obesity is by using a chart that calculates what's called the body mass index, or BMI, for short.

This chart, which shows the relationship between your height and weight, is based on the premise that above a certain level you are at greater risk for diseases like high blood pressure, diabetes, gout, certain cancers, gallbladder problems, sleep disorders, and arthritis.

This simple chart is valid for both men and women of all ages.

In this scheme, a woman who stands 5-foot 4½ is overweight if she weighs more than 147 pounds. She becomes obese if she weighs over 175.

A man 5-foot 10 is considered obese if he weighs more than 209 pounds.

Use the chart on page 30 to figure out your BMI. To determine your body mass index, locate your height in the far left column of the chart. Look along the line of weight boxes to the right of your height and find the weight box closest to your weight.

Next, look down at the very bottom of the column that your weight box is in. That's your BMI.

What does this number mean?

Simple:

You are considered normal weight if your body mass index is below 25.

You are considered overweight if your body mass index is above 26.

You are considered obese if your body mass index is above 30.

THE SKINNY ON OBESITY

The word obesity derives from the Latin for overeating. But overeating doesn't entirely explain obesity.

Inactivity doesn't, either, although the Center for Health Statistics estimates that seven in ten people don't exercise enough and four out of ten don't exercise at all!

This sounds like the usual view of obesity—that the obese eat too much and exercise too little, doesn't it?

But there is growing recognition, not just in the medical commu-

Body Mass Index (BMI) Chart

Height	Weight in Pounds											
4'11"	94	99	104	109	114	119	124	128	133	138	143	148
5'0"	97	102	107	112	117	122	128	133	138	143	148	153
5'1"	100	106	111	116	121	127	132	137	143	148	153	158
5'2"	103	108	114	119	124	130	136	142	147	153	158	164
5'3"	107	113	118	124	130	135	141	146	152	158	163	169
5'4"	110	115	121	127	133	138	145	151	157	163	169	174
5'5"	114	120	126	132	138	144	150	156	162	168	174	180
5'6"	118	124	130	136	143	149	155	161	167	173	179	185
5'7"	121	127	134	140	147	153	159	166	172	178	185	191
5'8"	124	130	137	143	150	156	164	171	177	184	190	197
5'9"	128	135	141	148	155	162	169	176	182	189	196	203
5'10"	133	139	146	153	160	167	174	181	188	195	202	209
5'11"	135	143	150	157	164	171	179	186	193	200	207	215
BMI	19	20	21	22	23	24	25	26	27	28	29	30

nity but even by the government, that obesity is not merely the result of lifestyle choices. It's a true medical problem. And the single most important factor leading to this radical rethinking is the discovery of obesity genes.

If the body has actual genes that control body fat, then being obese is a function of a body system gone wrong, just like any other disease, and not the result of poor eating or exercising habits. There is no longer any doubt that weight gain in humans, like weight loss, is controlled by genes.

There is a significant difference between the two, though: Weight loss is governed far more by genetics than weight gain is. This simple physiological fact explains a simple observation we've all known for years: It's easier to gain weight than lose weight!

Scientists estimate that genes play about a 50 percent role in your weight gain, which means that half of your body weight is determined by genes and not by overeating, eating incorrectly, exercising too little, etc.

But genes play a much larger role—sometimes as much as 90 percent—in weight loss!

The genetic discrepancy between weight gain and weight loss is best evidenced when we take a closer look at the number one risk factor for weight gain: the food supply.

The more food that is available, the greater your chances of gaining weight. For example, most of Central Africa has major food shortages. People living there habitually subsist at near-starvation levels and are among the thinnest populations on the globe.

Yet, when people emigrate from Africa to the United States, where there is an abundant food supply, they are just as likely to become overweight as other Americans.

You would think that it would be easier for someone new to the obesity game to lose weight than, say, someone who has a long and strong family history of obesity.

Not so!

Not even thousands of years of exposing their genes to a meager

If You're Overweight, Uncle Sam Wants You!

The 7-Minute Miracle can help fatten your wallet while slimming your hot spots. It's true! This could be the first weight-loss book to make you money.

Because I'm going to let you in on a secret: The U.S. government is now offering a tax break for medical costs incurred for the treatment of overweight or obesity. This deduction can even be taken for a few years prior!

If you qualify, you are allowed to deduct weight-loss treatments as a medical expense if your total medical deductions exceed 7.5 percent of your gross adjusted income. Your deductions must be itemized. If you want to get credit for previous years' treatments and expenses, you must file an amended return for the tax year in question. Do I sound like an accountant?

I'm the son of one!

Under the new tax plan you qualify for the tax write-off if your BMI is above 26, but this cutoff may change.

Your doctor should receive the new federal guidelines soon. It's not entirely clear yet what weight-loss treatments are covered, but the initial press release specifically mentioned that cosmetic and commercial

supply of food can protect them against the onslaught of a readily available food supply. Once excess fat gets stored in your fat cells, your weight control genes take over.

Yet, even if you are obese, The 7-Minute Miracle allows you to overcome this genetic stranglehold. Conceptually, if you are obese, you simply have larger fat deposits at the five hot spots and other body sites than your thinner counterparts.

OBESITY'S SECRET WEAPON

Your size, if you are obese, can be your secret weapon, too.

That's because the more body fat you have, the more you lose. And, in general, the more body fat you have, the easier it is to shed pounds.

weight-loss programs and diet foods are not covered (which shows how effective they are!), nor is joining a gym to "improve the taxpayer's appearance, general health, and sense of well-being." Nor will things like liposuction, massage, spas, etc., be covered.

But the government apparently will allow deductions for plans supervised by doctors, including behavior therapy and weight-loss medications. Eventually insurers, including Medicare, may get in on the action, too.

If you have questions, speak to your accountant or go to www.irs.gov, the Internal Revenue Service's web site. I also suggest that you try the excellent web site of the not-for-profit agency Obesity Association of America, headed by the well-known weight-loss expert Dr. George Atkinson.

What's most eye-opening and revolutionary about this shift in national health policy is that those little pieces of DNA in your fat cells got all those suits in Washington excited enough to change the tax code.

That's gene power!

This is based on fundamental thermodynamics.

It goes like this:

More body fat means a larger body surface area. The larger your body surface area, the higher your metabolism. The higher your metabolism, the easier it is to burn fat.

Next time someone asks you, "Who has a higher metabolism: a hummingbird or an elephant?" you should know the answer right away: the elephant, by a mile!

Following The 7-Minute Miracle allows you to burn fat quicker than a thinner person. Having larger fat deposits, though, means that it takes longer to see the results, so give it time.

Remember: If you are obese, your size is your secret weapon.

Use it.

CRACKING YOUR GENETIC CODE

Each brick of fat in your personal pyramid is placed there by genes. These tiny, spiral staircase-shaped strands of DNA are found in each cell of your body, including your fat cells. Genes are your body's blueprint, ordaining which proteins—the building blocks of your body—are to be constructed. Genes are also responsible for your body's day-to-day activities, from how your heart beats to the way your body digests food.

To break out from your own pyramid and lose weight from a particular spot, you have to redirect the same energy that the body uses to keep the entire pyramid standing to one spot. Our goal is to take the same genes that push your fat *into* fat cells and make them push your fat *out* of fat cells. That's the radical new idea behind the 7-Minute Miracle Genetic Body Sculpting Plan.

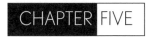
STEP AWAY FROM THE SCALE!

It took five thousand years of organized medicine before someone even thought that weighing humans had some scientific merit. And it was yet another 300 years before people mustered the courage to bring the scale into their homes and actually weigh themselves!

Around 1930 the Continental Scale Works company introduced the first bathroom scale in Chicago. It was called the Health-O-Meter, a name that's still around.

One custom that started back then endures: We like to weigh ourselves in the inner sanctum of the most private of private areas, the bathroom. With the door locked, of course.

I tell you all of this not because I think it's time that you knew the history of the scale, but because I believe it's time that you make your scale history.

Face it. If you dream of a more streamlined body, then you know that looking good in the mirror is far more satisfying than seeing

Help! I'm a Scale-o-holic!

If having extra-large hips or thighs is enough to drive you up a wall, then worrying about how much a scale says you weigh is more then enough to drive you over a wall.

I remember Denise S., a 40-year-old paralegal who told me that her bathroom scale was making her crazy. It started with her early-morning weigh-in. If the number on the scale didn't match what she thought it should be, Denise would curse, kick the scale and eat nothing that day until her willpower gave out, usually about five hours later.

With any luck, though, the number on the scale would mesh better with the number in her brain at one of her five to ten afternoon and evening weigh-ins.

I advised her to get rid of the scale. She couldn't. She said that this particular scale had it in for her and that she was going to beat it. As a compromise, we struck a deal. For a one-week test period, she would give the scale to her friend around the corner to hold for her. I figured that since it was the middle of winter, she would be less likely to retrieve it from there, as opposed to from a neighbor next door.

Three days into our little experiment, I received a call from the emergency room of the local hospital, letting me know that Denise was there, getting a cast for a broken wrist.

She evidently slipped on the black ice in front of the house of her friend around the corner. She went there to weigh herself, at 11:30 at night! In 18 degree weather!

Trust me on this one: It's just not worth it, folks.

some arbitrary number on a scale. That's why I want you to put your scale away, for a while. You don't need it to spot reduce. From this point on, your focus should be on size and proportion, not weight.

Don't get hung up on the whole pounds thing. You are not a hunk of beef measured by weight alone. Certainly, you will lose pounds by following The 7-Minute Miracle, but slimming your body contours, and fitting into smaller dress sizes and tighter pants are what you're really after, right?

SEEING IS BELIEVING

Home scales and most doctors' scales aren't sensitive enough to measure spot fat loss anyway, so why bother? What your thighs and hips weigh is not as important as how trim and fit they are.

Common sense and simple observation are the tools you use to measure progress, not the number of pounds lost. But if you are the type who needs to see an objective measurement, then get out the old 99-cent tape measure, and start keeping a spot reducing log.

Every few days, measure your own hot spot, whether it's your upper arms, belly, hips, butt, or thighs. As it shrinks, record your results.

And if that's not enough number-crunching for you, start paying attention to your new, smaller dress and pants size. Count as you change belt loops. Count the compliments you get.

Count your smiles as you shrink down your most troublesome body part.

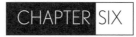

CHAPTER SIX

CHOOSING YOUR
DEFINING MOMENT

If you're still not sure which is more important—building bigger muscles or burning more fat—just turn on the TV on any given Sunday in autumn. The average National Football League lineman weighs close to 300 pounds. You don't need a giant projection TV to see that many of them—as Homer Simpson once put it—don't have six-pack abs, they have kegs.

But don't get fooled. What you see is not what you get.

Under all that blubber lies a firm foundation of super-strong, super-developed abdominal muscles. I have performed physicals on many of these behemoths before they left for training camp. I assure you that even with their abs smothered in fat, these players can do more sit-ups than you, me, and your two best friends put together.

What on earth can make such huge muscles disappear like they were part of a bad David Copperfield trick? Fat.

To see your muscles again, you need to dig them out from under the fat, and define them. Freeing your hips, thighs, belly, arms, and butt muscles from layers of fat lets them stand out and bask in all their defined glory.

Muscles devoid of fat are defined, highly visible, and aesthetically pleasing. Muscles bathed in fat are ill-defined and barely visible, if not totally hidden under your skin.

The difference between muscle visibility and muscle invisibility at any of the five hot spots can be as little as an eighth of an inch of fat. What makes little difference, though, is how big and well developed your muscles are in these areas.

This concept is frequently lost on exercise experts who mistakenly lump the terms muscular development and muscular definition together. They are not the same.

Here's why:

Muscular development is based entirely on muscle tissue growth because—even if we pump more iron than Arnold Schwarzenegger—we can't increase the number of muscles we have. We can only increase muscle size.

Muscles get bigger when you make them work and feed them enough nutrients, the process known as hypertrophy. Muscles that aren't worked, don't grow. They stagnate. If they aren't used over periods of time, they get smaller, or atrophy (Greek for not fed), the opposite of hypertrophy.

SHOULD YOU JOIN THE RESISTANCE?

The apple that crowned Sir Isaac Newton did you a big favor. Lore has it that the fruit that bonked Newton's skull enabled him to figure out gravity. Gravity not only keeps your feet on the ground, it keeps your muscles fit, too. Whenever you move, your muscles are stimulated to grow because they are fighting the downward force of gravity. Even such routine activities as getting out of bed, combing your hair, and eating make your muscles grow.

Astronauts and Atrophy

When John Glenn returned from his first voyage in space manning Friendship 7 in 1962, he could barely walk for days because his leg muscles were so shriveled from confinement in the tiny space capsule.

The space people got smarter over the years, and when Glenn returned from his historic, 9-day 1998 space mission aboard the space shuttle Discovery, he got his "earth legs" back almost immediately.

His secret was to exercise for short periods of time, keeping blood flowing to his leg muscles. This was based on the earlier work of scientists like Dr. Laurence E. Morehouse, director of the Human Performance Laboratory at the University of California, Los Angeles, and a NASA consultant, who found that quick spurts (as little as 5 minutes' worth) of intense physical activity is enough to combat muscle atrophy.

It's a valuable lesson that applies to those of us who are earth-bound, as well as astronauts. In fact, it's one of the keys to The 7-Minute Miracle. More about that later.

But muscles grow to the max by any work or play activity that forces them to contract against resistance. For instance, weightlifting and gymnastics favor muscular development much more than walking because they force your muscles to contract against a load. Continued habitual weight training makes your muscles bigger and, usually, stronger.

There are many reasons why you would want bigger and stronger muscles. Increased overall physical and mental health and perhaps longevity head a long list of wonderful benefits bestowed by having developed muscles. Not to mention greater sex appeal and a shot in the arm to self-esteem.

But as with any biological process, there are limits to how much muscle you can develop. Not everyone who lifts weights, for example, develops enough muscle to gain the health benefits as advertised.

Years ago, I worked out at Dan Lurie's gym in Brooklyn, around the corner from Barbra Streisand's High School, Erasmus Hall. For you trivia buffs, Dan Lurie, a local fitness pioneer, was Circus Dan the Muscle Man on the CBS-TV show The Big Top in the mid-1950's. (And for you serious trivia buffs, the Head Clown on The Big Top was none other than Ed McMahon. But I digress.)

To recruit new members, the gym hired attractive young women, outfitted them in micro-minis and white go-go boots and sent them out to the street below. Their mission was to comb the area around the gym to entice young men to come upstairs for a gym look-see. If they liked what they saw, they would join on the spot.

I remember one "catch of the day," a thin-as-a-wet-Q-tip wiseguy, who came by for the tour while I was working out. He wanted to join, but some pictures hanging above the mirrors were giving him second thoughts.

What he was looking at were photos of the bodybuilding stars of the day: Arnold Schwarzenegger, Franco Columbo, Chuck Sipes, Lou Ferrigno, and the gym's own Mr. America, Kenny Hall.

Pointing to the pictures, the new kid on the block said, "I want to put on a little more muscle, but, geez, I don't want to look like these guys."

"Oh, don't worry about that," I assured him, "One thing I promise: You will *never* look like them."

I still get a kick out of this story.

I mean, really, here was this walking toothpick worrying about turning into a world-class bodybuilder, overnight. World-class body-builders are a rare, rare, breed. And for good reason: It turns out that building muscle and strength are also genetic!

No matter how much you exercise, no matter how many weights you lift, unless you have the right genes, you cannot get appreciably bigger or stronger. Science has shown that your genes make putting on lots of muscle a daunting, lifelong endeavor, reserved for a special few.

Anyway, having all the muscle in the world still won't make you a Mr. or Ms. Universe if those muscles are cloaked in fat. Define the muscles that you have by getting rid of extra fat and you're in business.

Fortunately, trimming away the fat and defining muscle is a lot easier than developing muscle. That works out great for you, because defining—not developing—muscle is where it's at if you want to lose any of your hot spots.

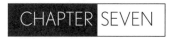
HITTING THE SPOT: A NEW APPROACH TO WEIGHT LOSS

In America these days, there's no question that we're living large. The National Institutes of Health estimates that more than half—61 percent—of Americans over age 20 are considered overweight.

To help put things in perspective, the average male Civil War soldier weighed less than 150 pounds. His male Desert Storm counterpart, 140 years later, weighed almost 35 pounds more!

If dreaming about losing your oversized thighs, hips, belly, butt, or arms has been easier than actually doing it, you are hardly alone. Not by a long shot.

Nearly everyone, no matter what they weigh, has a mound of local fat that they would love to part company with, but can't. That's why a recent survey shows that 55 percent of Americans are on diets.

The inability of most overweight persons to bring their weight down to levels even close to what health experts and insurance companies refer to as their "ideal body weight" has fueled a new trend in weight loss—that of opting for spot reduction.

Lately, I've noticed that my patients are more likely to ask, "Doctor, how wide should my waist be?" or "How can I make the back of my arms smaller?" than, "Doctor, how much should I weigh?"

I'll bet you experienced the same phenomenon right in your own bedroom.

It goes something like this. Instead of a significant other asking you, "Honey, do I look fat in these pants?" they may ask, "Honey, do these pants make my tush look big?"

Questions like this one reflect a fundamental shift in attitude regarding weight loss in this country. We are finally coming to our senses, thank goodness, by paying less attention to arbitrary numbers on a scale and scaling down our weight loss goals. More and more people are making spot weight loss a priority over total body weight loss, which is far more difficult for all the reasons I've discussed in the previous chapters.

Over the long run, genes and certain brain chemicals control body weight. Together, they create a narrow range of body weight that we are essentially stuck with. Losing a lot of weight outside of this range to reach an "ideal" body weight is difficult because your body is genetically dead-set against it.

Now you understand why celebrities, armed with entourages of personal chefs and personal trainers, can't do it, and neither can we regular folk.

A PINCH IN TIME

The 7-Minute Miracle doesn't put pressure on you to go from overweight to svelte, overnight. Instead, I want you to target one specific area of your body—the hot spot that bothers you the most, whether it's your belly, butt, thighs, hips, or arms—and focus your weight-loss efforts on slimming it down. Guaranteed: It will work, and you will feel better about yourself.

Each of us, if we're totally honest with ourselves, has one particular area of our body we'd really like to improve. If you want to find out if you have fat to burn, just try the simple, time-tested, pinch test.

Take a hard-cover book and, with a ruler, measure out three-quarters of an inch in page thickness. Pinch the pages with your thumb and forefinger, so you get used to what three-quarters of an inch feels like.

Now, let's see how you stack up.

Using the same thumb and forefinger, gently pinch the body spot in question, be it your belly, butt, thighs, hips, or arms. If you can pinch three-quarters of an inch or more, then you've spotted a problem.

Any stubborn, fatty body part that won't slim down, no matter what you try, can drive you batty. To see if your spot fat deposits are playing mind and body games with you, take this personal spot fat quiz.

PERSONAL SPOT FAT QUIZ

1. Do you try to hide particular body parts by wearing camouflaging colors and styles of clothing?

Yes_____   No_____

2. Do you feel that an oversized body part makes you less attractive?

Yes_____   No_____

3. Do you believe that "Everything I eat goes to" a specific body part like your hips?

Yes_____   No_____

4. Does a single body part prevent you from fitting into tighter jeans?

Yes_____   No_____

5. Are you overly sensitive to comments made about a specific body part?

                                        Yes_____   No_____

If you answered "yes" to any of these five questions, it's an easy bet that a body part or two has gotten the best of you.

REVEAL, DON'T CONCEAL

That only a dab of extra fat can lower your self-esteem demonstrates the power that spot fat can wield over us. If you wear "baggies" to hide a pair of extra-wide hips, or sweat it out in long-sleeved shirts right smack in the middle of summer because you're self-conscious about flabby arms, you may be part of the great American cover-up: dressing to conceal your least-liked body part.

But no matter how good you are at covering up, you can't render your hips, belly, thighs, butt, or arms invisible. Take the old "sweater tied loosely around the waist to hide the tush" trick. Some trick. It really draws attention away from your backside, doesn't it?

It's time for an about-face. It's time to get rid of your extra fat, and stop hiding it. I want you to be proud of your body, to reveal it, not conceal it.

What about you? Do you feel that you have lost control over a particular body part?

Many patients tell me that they have.

Listen to Julia R., a 25-year-old real estate agent from Connecticut, who, near tears at her initial consultation, said, "I'm successful at my job, my marriage is great, my family is healthy. The only thing that I can't seem to control are these hips."

She then stood up and in one motion, as if curtseying, bent forward, pointed to her hips with both hands, rolled her eyes upward, and sat down again.

Feeling like you're not in control can be a real bummer. But spot reducing allows you to regain control because it's easier to conquer a smaller area than a larger one. It's a lot more rewarding, too.

That's why losing inches captivates you more than pounds lost. That's why going down a dress or pants size is far more satisfying than chasing a number on a scale.

Now that you've identified your personal hot spot, it's time to start back taking control. I'll show you how, with The 7-Minute Miracle Genetic Body Sculpting Plan.

THE GENETIC BODY SCULPTING PLAN

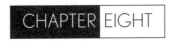

CHAPTER EIGHT

ADRENALINE: THE SPARK THAT IGNITES FAT-BURNING

Day in and night out, whether you are asleep or awake, your heart pumps blood to every organ of your body. And nature sees to it that the fat and muscle at each of your hot spots are fed by the same veins and arteries. This means that when blood flows to your abdominal muscles, for example, the adjacent belly fat is nourished by the same blood.

The same is true for your hips, butt, thighs, and arms. They each share the same blood supply with their neighboring fat, like good blood brothers and sisters should. When you exercise, blood flow to your muscles increases, proportional to the amount of exertion. The more you exercise your muscles, the more blood they receive. Research indicates that muscles activate unused capillaries, the tiny blood vessels that connect arteries and veins.

So exercising any of your hot spots draws extra blood there. But there's exercise, and there's vigorous exercise. They are not the same.

Of Mice and Muscle

Do you hate mice? Not so fast. They're strong little critters, plus they have excellent taste. I should know. One once gnawed through a wooden hutch in my dining room to get at a gold-leafed box of Godiva chocolates.

So it shouldn't come as a complete surprise that the word "muscle" comes from the Latin word for mouse. To the Romans, contracting muscles—especially the biceps—reminded them of little mice scrambling under the skin.

The whole Mighty Mouse cartoon thing makes more sense now, right?

But the bond between muscle and mouse is deeper than their common word origin. The genetic research that finally cracked the fat-gene code was done on these furry guys first. Lucky for us, many of the same weight-loss genes found in mice were found in humans, too.

I find it interesting that the scientists who conducted the research could make mice miss meals and deprive themselves of sleep and even sex. But you know what the mice *didn't* do? They didn't lift weights.

Now, I'll admit that the thought of buff, ranting rodents lifting miniature barbells, strutting their stuff on the beach, is good for a few giggles. But there's a point here. To lose weight, the mice didn't take up weight training.

Neither should you.

The difference in the effect on your blood flow between weight lifting and the routines you'll find in The 7-Minute Miracle Workout is similar to the difference between an idyllic stream and raging, white-water rapids.

When in full gear, exercising muscles start pumping blood themselves, giving your heart a powerful boost and sending extra blood to adjacent fat deposits. So forget pumping iron, you want to pump blood.

Why? Because the blood that your muscles pump is special. It's rich in epinephrine, the king of all fat burners.

THE ADRENALINE CONNECTION

Epinephrine is your primary stress hormone. When your brain perceives a threat, it activates your primal "fight-or-flight" response, which includes pumping epinephrine into your system to heighten awareness and readiness. From the Greek meaning "above the kidneys," epinephrine is manufactured by paired adrenal glands above your kidneys. You probably know epinephrine by its more common name, adrenaline, the term we will use.

Adrenaline causes your heart to pound and your pulse and breathing rate to soar whenever you are confronted by stress, like when speaking in public. Strenuous exercise is also a type of physical stress and that's why muscles in motion attract adrenaline like kicking legs in the movie *Jaws* attracted the great shark.

Since muscle and fat are connected by the same arteries, some of this adrenaline passes from muscle to nearby fat. The hormone also reaches fat cells via nerves that originate in the adrenal glands.

That two separate pathways evolved for adrenaline to reach your fat cells attests to its importance as your body's chief short-term, fat-burning hormone. Adrenaline, alone, has the power to melt away the fat on your belly, butt, thighs, hips, or arms by giving fat cells the jolt they need to get moving.

FANNING THE FAT-BURNING FLAMES

As Bruce Springsteen once said, "You can't start a fire without a spark." That's true for love, and it's equally true for fat-burning.

And when it comes to fat-burning, adrenaline is the spark.

Your fat cells, you'll recall from Part One, have an on-off switch on the outside known as the G-protein. If you want to burn fat, this

Walk On By

Brenda W., a 29-year-old mother of three, once told me that one of the perks of owning a nail salon is that after the last customer leaves the shop, she gets to read the magazines left lying around.

One evening, she went through a national weekly with a four-letter name that rhymes with the kind of work that Marcel Marceau does. A cover story on fitness advised readers that if they were looking for one good overall exercise, they should take up walking.

It sounded good to Brenda, so she went out and bought hot new cross-trainers and a cool, all-weather training suit in bold orange. Away she went, determined to shrink her tush.

Next time I saw her, Brenda told me: "I'm toast. No more exercise. Six weeks straight—rain, hangover, migraine, whatever—I dragged myself out of bed and walked my butt off at Westwood High's track. Or so I thought.

"I couldn't have walked anything off 'cause my butt is still as big as a Mack truck." (Don't hold back, Brenda, tell us how you really feel!)

Brenda was angry not only at herself, but also at her choice of exercise: walking. I hear a lot of my patients playing this exercise blame-game. The problem is that they, Brenda included, use exercise like Ginsu knives: on a trial basis.

They're willing to give things a try for a few weeks, but if they don't see results quickly, they feel cheated and disgusted.

Get real.

Walking is just doing what it's programmed to do when it comes to spot reducing: nothing. You can't walk your butt off, because walking won't give you an adrenaline rush. It's that simple.

switch must be turned on to send the message to the enzyme lipase inside the cell that it's time for fat to hit the highway.

If the circumstances are right, adrenaline can turn on the G-protein switch and spark the fat-burning process—lipolysis—to life. It's like lightning was to the two-story contraption Dr. Frankenstein used to bring his creature to life.

Without adrenaline, fat cells take a lifelong siesta.

So it's pretty simple: What you need is a way to get adrenaline to the exact clump of fat cells you choose to spark the fat-burning process there.

You need look no further than your own muscles.

By exercising the muscles that lie directly beneath your unwanted fat, you increase local blood flow, simultaneously transporting fat-pulverizing adrenaline to the same spot.

It certainly makes sense, doesn't it?

Let's use your thighs as an example. Exercising them increases blood flow to your thigh muscles. This blood, loaded with adrenaline, then gets pumped from your thigh muscles to your thigh fat, triggering the process to begin dumping fat from your fat cells there.

This exact scenario should play out at your hips, belly, backsides, or arms, too, if that's the area you choose. It should, but don't dust off your old gym membership card just yet.

Doesn't all this sound too familiar to suit you? Haven't you done sit-ups and crunches in the past, which theoretically should have transported adrenaline to your midsection fat, without noticing any difference?

Didn't a women's or men's magazine article—or 60—promise that all those side bends you tried would take care of your love handles? What happened?

Somewhere along the line, they forgot to tell you about the adrenaline barrier.

STORMING THE ADRENALINE BARRIER

In a perfect world, any exercise should help you spot reduce. In the real world, most can't, because they can't trigger the fat-burning process. The reason? Your body has a natural resistance to giving adrenaline easy access to your fat cells.

I call it the adrenaline barrier.

Each of you has a genetically determined adrenaline barrier that can block you from losing weight at the five hot spots. This helps explain why some people burn fat quicker than others.

Not a day goes by without someone telling me about friends, relatives, or coworkers who lose weight much quicker than they do, as if some mystical force divines their separate weight-loss fortunes.

It's not mystical; it's biological. It's your adrenaline barrier at work.

Over the long haul, especially if you become less active as you age, your body's ability to manufacture and handle adrenaline declines. This explains why certain body functions like fat-burning, heart rate, and pulse slow over the years.

It's as if nature lessens its expectations of us as we age.

To smash through your adrenaline barrier, you need an adrenaline rush. That's what you get when you exercise in a way that concentrates enough adrenaline in a particular area to overcome the local fat-burning blockade at your belly, butt, thighs, hips, and arms.

But first, let's talk about how *not* to exercise. Because as much as I hate to be the one to break the news to you, almost everything you've been told about exercise and weight loss is wrong.

DON'T SPREAD YOURSELF THIN!

To lose your spot fat, you don't have to lift weights. Nor do you have to walk or ride a bicycle, and you certainly don't have to buy a glider, strider, trainer, or treadmill. The hot new workout trends, like kick boxing, power yoga, or Pilates? Like we say in my old Brooklyn neighborhood: fuhgedaboudit!

All of these techniques, along with traditional weight-loss exercises like tennis and stationary bicycling, share one fatal spot-reducing flaw: By definition, these activities require that you exercise many muscle groups at the same time.

That's their hook! For years, we've been told that these types of global exercises give you the most bang for your exercise buck.

When you walk, for instance, the power comes from your legs, and you swing your arms for balance while your spinal erector muscles tense and fight gravity to keep your back and neck upright.

The problem is a simple logistics one.

By using so many muscles at once, you spread blood flow too thinly throughout your body, so that no one area receives more blood or adrenaline than another.

That's why these exercises are ineffective as local fat burners. They dilute adrenaline instead of concentrating it to the hot spot where you need it. The result: You never break through the adrenaline barrier, so you get frustrated and stop exercising.

Ninety-five percent of my patients freely admit that they don't exercise. This incredible number of no-shows indicates that something is wrong out there in exercise land.

Specific body part exercises, like sit-ups or crunches for abs, won't give you an adrenaline rush, either, even though they use fewer muscle groups. Crunches are certainly great ab muscle builders, but they don't channel enough adrenaline to the deeper and often hidden muscle fibers of your abdomen to be effective local fat-burners.

Intuitively, you realize that the more muscle fibers you have pumping blood, the more adrenaline will be on hand to hit the hot spot. To get an adrenaline rush, you need to exercise the maximum amount of muscle fibers available at each hot spot, something that even sit-ups or crunches can't do for you.

So before you do your next set of sit-ups, sit up and listen: No matter which gym you join, no matter how many personal trainers you hire or which supplements and equipment you try, without the adrenaline rush—without getting enough adrenaline to the exact spot you need to—you won't succeed in spot reducing.

This is true whether you work out for 20 minutes or 2 hours.

Twenty minutes? Two hours?

Now here's the really good news: It won't take anywhere near that long to successfully spot reduce, *if* you work out the right way. In fact, in less time than it takes to listen to Don McLean's American Pie or Led Zeppelin's Stairway to Heaven on the Oldies station, you can slim down and reshape your body.

That's the promise of The 7-Minute Miracle Workout. But be forewarned: This isn't like any other workout you've ever tried. It's intense. But you can do it. And unlike the other workouts you've tried, it works.

Andy Warhol predicted that, sometime in the future, we'd all be famous for 15 minutes. But I'm telling you that in less than half that time, you can be *fabulous*.

All it takes is 7 minutes a day.

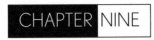

CHAPTER NINE

STOP COUNTING, AND MAKE YOUR EXERCISE COUNT

I'm sitting here reading a couple of fitness magazines, and I must confess: The cover lines sure sound enticing:

Hips and Thighs of Envy

Super Chest Blasting

Washboard Abdominals in Three Weeks

What I forgot to mention is that the magazines I'm reading are *Strength & Health* and *Muscular Development*—from 1962!

We've been falling for the same empty promises and doing the same routines for more than 40 years. Only the equipment has changed—pec decks and fly machines for the chest, leg press and abductor machines for legs.

Been there, done that!

And we're still stuck with the same old set-and-rep counting mindset. You know the one: "Do two sets of 10 repetitions."

I wonder how many billion sets and reps have been counted out in gyms since those articles appeared 40 years ago?

"One, two, three, kick."

"One two, three, pull."

"One two, three, bend."

Been there, counted that.

It's time to stop counting, and start making our exercise count. It's time to start reducing.

CLAMPING DOWN ON FAT

Our strategy is simple.

We've got five separate mini-workouts for you, each targeting a specific hot spot: the belly, butt, thighs, hips, or arms. You choose the one you want to whittle down first. Each 7-Minute Miracle Workout isolates only those muscles that pump the most adrenaline to your hot spot, allowing you to smash through your adrenaline barrier there.

They were developed by going to the pros: the researchers who work with adrenaline in the laboratory. They know how to get the most fat out of fat cells. That's their job.

One of the chief research methods scientists use to study fat cells is the microdialysis technique. This is a temporary surgical procedure performed on the abdomen because it offers the easiest access, but the results are valid for your thighs, hips, arms, and butt.

Using volunteers, hopefully paid ones, researchers implant (ooh!) a tiny tube called a microcatheter into abdominal fat right beneath the skin surface. This opens a direct line to fat cells.

The scientists then clamp off blood flow so they can measure what goes in and out of the fat cells. The cells manufacture many substances, but what interests us most are gene products. These are molecules made by fat-cell genes in response to exercise, different kinds of foods, and other environmental stimulants.

You can actually measure what goes on inside your fat cells. You can see if there really is a difference between eating a Snickers candy bar or a salad. You can measure if your fat cells are at all impressed by that treadmill you just bought.

ACTIVATING YOUR FAT CELLS

To test the effect of any substance on your fat cells, scientists inject the compound in question directly into the abdominal catheter and wait. For example, should the adrenaline from exercise or protein from a steak stimulate fat cells, they create positive feedback, nudging the DNA of fat cell genes to make messenger RNA (ribonucleic acid), a gene product that's a sure sign of fat cell activation and potential fat loss. Messenger RNA, or mRNA, is then measured and quantified.

If no mRNA is detected, then the fat cells are in negative feedback mode, the cell is not activated, and there is no fat loss. In other words, siesta time.

By the way, the clamp technique also was used to determine which foods activate weight-loss genes and which don't. That research is the basis of The 7-Minute Miracle Meal Plan, which we'll get to later in this part of the book.

Through these scientific tests, we learned that the secret to local fat-burning is fat cell activation.

To activate your fat cells, they must be exposed to a continuous flow of adrenaline-rich blood. Fat cells exposed to a lowered, or stop-and-go, pattern of adrenaline are not as highly activated. And the research showed that there is an optimum time for the continuous flow of adrenaline-rich blood.

It's exactly 7 minutes.

Once you know which muscles best move adrenaline-rich blood to your hot spot, you're set. The trick is finding the right exercises to work those muscles at a level that keeps the adrenaline and blood pumping.

You'll find those exercises in The 7-Minute Miracle Workout. But first, there are three keys you will need to unlock the full fat-burning potential of the exercises.

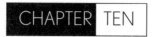

CHAPTER TEN

CSI: THE SECRETS TO A FAT-BURNING WORKOUT

What some exercise programs do to you is a crime. So it's time to call in CSI. No, not Crime Scene Investigation. I'm talking about the three keys that transform exercise into a spot-reducing blast:

- Combining
- Sequencing
- Intensity

No matter which hot spot troubles you most, these three keys transform a regular workout into a fat cell-activating and spot-reducing one. If you consistently apply these principles each time you do your 7-minute workout, you'll be guaranteed to get that adrenaline pumping and send those fat cells running. The principles of CSI set The 7-Minute Miracle apart from any other exercise program you've tried. So let's bring them in for a lineup, one at a time.

Hip Pointers

Before you begin this or any exercise program, there are certain basics.

Should you have any questions regarding your physical condition or your ability to participate in an exercise program, talk to your physician. Be sure to obtain medical clearance before any exercise if you

- are pregnant
- are breastfeeding
- have a chronic medical condition, like cardiovascular disease, arthritis, or diabetes
- take medication for a chronic condition like high blood pressure

In this day and age, anyone over age 40 who hasn't exercised on a regular basis should have a complete physical examination and a stress test, if indicated.

Medical issues aside, don't forget to exercise common sense before you exercise your body.

- Never hold your breath when you exercise.
- Stop if you feel pain in any part of your body.
- Exercise in a room that has good air flow.
- Don't exercise on a full stomach.
- Have plenty of water on hand.
- Dress so that your skin can breathe. No rubber suits.
- Avoid hot, humid rooms.

COMBINING: STRENGTH IN NUMBERS

Once I knew the science, I needed to figure out how to turn it into an exercise program that worked. I started with a reliable anatomical textbook to delineate the main blood vessels supplying both the muscles and fat of each hot spot. Most anatomical texts do not depict abnormal adult-sized fat pads. So I had to draw in my own. Then I traced out a grid of the blood vessels for each hot spot.

Next, I superimposed the grid on top of a kinesiology muscle map illustrating which muscles are involved in particular exercises. This allowed me to pick out only those muscles with the largest exposure to shared blood vessels with local fat deposits. These are the muscles that should pump the most blood and adrenaline to the fat pads and activate the fat cells there.

When I took a closer look at the muscle groups involved, it became clear that no one hot spot can be effectively covered by one exercise alone, or even two. No two exercises hit enough muscle fiber at each hot spot to get the necessary amount of adrenaline to the site.

The unique anatomical relationships forged by the fat cells, muscles, and blood vessels at each hot spot require three exercises per body part. The exercises I've chosen are designed to work all of the muscle groups of a hot spot in one 7-minute workout. Together, the three exercises create a synergistic adrenaline-concentrating effect by getting at most of the muscle fibers in an area, including the hidden ones that regular exercise doesn't hit.

I ran the plan by dozens of trainers and bodybuilders. I learned that everyone has their own "best exercise" candidates for each hot spot.

With safety and effectiveness in mind, I sought movements with the least injury potential that could be done by anyone, regardless of age or physical prowess. I sure didn't want any that would require a degree in exercise physiology.

In the end, I've come up with three exercises per body part that burn the most fat at each hot spot, in the shortest amount of time. The three exercises for each body part combine to be stronger as local fat burners than they would be as individuals.

That's what exercise combining is all about: Combining three exercises that target each of the five hot spots and concentrate enough adrenaline to burn fat there.

But it's how you move from one exercise to the next that takes them to the next level.

SEQUENCING: THE 7-MINUTE SOLUTION
TO THE 20-MINUTE DILEMMA

Not long ago, at a local gym, I overheard a TV anchor ask his personal trainer after doing a set of side bends for his love handles, "Why do I have to do ten reps? My old trainer said that seven reps are enough. Ten reps just tears the muscle down"

The trainer, looking unfazed, apparently having fielded this question before, answered nonchalantly: "Ten reps are better for definition. Seven reps or less bulk you up. You should do more sets."

"But my old trainer always said that too many sets fatigues the muscle, stunting its growth," countered the anchorman.

"Not so," the trainer shot back. "Muscles tend to grow with more sets."

I was dying inside. I've already told you to stop counting, and start making your exercise count. So let me say it again: No more sets and reps. They're killing your workouts and your chance for spot reducing.

Many patients find the entire rep/set system to be stifling and intimidating because it robs them of spontaneity. Who would play basketball, if counting every dribble was part of the rules, or tennis, if you had to count each hit?

Stop counting!

Reps, and sets in particular, lose their relevancy because spot-reducing success is based on continuous exercise for 7 minutes without stopping. Sets, by definition, mean that you must stop moving, take a rest, then resume once more.

Think about what happens inside your body under stop-and-go conditions. Each pause slows blood flow, changing the pattern of availability of adrenaline, lulling your fat cells back to sleep.

Your fat cells respond best to the constant blood flow instigated by 7 minutes of continuous muscular exercise This brings us to the second transforming element of spot reducing: exercise sequencing.

Exercise sequencing means that we do the three exercises one after another in one 7-minute stint without counting sets or reps. Moving continuously from one exercise to another has one great advantage: It lets you overcome the arch enemy of any single form of continuous exercise: fatigue. Moving continuously lets you enter the aerobic zone.

Texas's Dr. Kenneth Cooper, the father of aerobics (he coined the word) is big on continuous exercise. On the basis of earlier research, he concluded that 20 minutes of continuous exercise is the minimum for the body to enter a fat-burning mode as it switches from carbohydrates to fats for muscle fuel.

Dr. Cooper envisioned millions of Americans staying in shape by doing at least 20 minutes of exercises like running or rowing. But running or rowing for 2 minutes is tough; 20 minutes is torture. That's why so few of us belong to track clubs, and why rowing regattas are never going to be confused with the World Series.

To paraphrase the old cartoon character Pogo, when it comes to the aerobic movement, we have met the enemy, and he is us. We never even reach the 20-minute minimum because we get fatigued too rapidly to enter the fat-burning, aerobic zone.

The 7-Minute Miracle offers a way out of this dilemma.

By sequencing three separate exercises, you move one group of muscles until they get fatigued, then move on to another group, giving the first group a chance to recover. By the time you finish the third exercise, the first group of muscles is ready for you once more, and soon the second group will be, too.

Moving forcefully and at a good pace through the three exercises stimulates your heart, creating one terrific mini-aerobic, cardiovascular workout that specifically targets your chosen hot spot.

Moving seamlessly from the first movement to the second and on to the third, without breaking, powers adrenaline to the area you're working, whether it's your belly, butt, thighs, hips, or arms. It's a beautiful weight-loss symphony, in three movements.

INTENSITY: EXERCISING WITH ENTHUSIASM AND EFFORT

I tell my kids that if someone is doing a job and it looks easy, it's probably hard. It's the worker's enthusiasm, experience, and effort that make their job look easy.

What The 7-Minute Miracle doesn't ask of you in time, it demands in effort. To supercharge your workout, add the third transforming element: intensity.

People who talk while they exercise drive me bonkers. So do people who exercise while they talk!

When I see people reading the Wall Street Journal or watching CNN while on the stationary bike, I remember what my friend Amy said the

Stop Signs

Here are eight warning signs that you are overdoing it and should stop, rest, and seek medical attention:

1. severe shortness of breath
2. muscle cramps
3. coughing
4. chest pain
5. wheezing
6. chest tightness
7. dizziness
8. excessive perspiration

first time she waded out far from shore in the shallow Adriatic Sea, off the coast of Pescara, Italy, without even getting the top of her thighs wet: "There no water in this water!"

There's no exercise in this exercise.

If you're talking, you're not exercising The 7-Minute Miracle way. During The 7-Minute Miracle Workout, you shouldn't be able to talk! Nor would you want to. That's just going through the motions, doing your body a favor.

I say: *Never exercise as if you're doing your body a favor.*

Your body is doing *you* a favor. Inject enthusiasm and zeal into your workout.

THAT'S LIFE

I tell my patients that the dead all have one thing in common: They don't move. Life is movement. So when patients tell me that they're dead tired, I tell them they're only half right. To put life back into their lives, I remind them, they need to not only exercise, but to put life back into their exercise. To get intense.

So do you.

When you go through the motions, your body senses it. When you get intense, your body appreciates that as special. No matter how smart you are, your body is smarter. It can't be tricked into thinking it's working hard if it's not.

Which cues let you know that you are exercising with intensity? I told you that your body is trying to tell you something. Here's what it is.

Get your heart rate up. Sweat. Pant.

ON THE RIGHT TRACK

Imagine you're at your high school track.

Run the 100-yard dash. Okay, make believe that you are running the 100-yard dash. How would you feel afterwards? Would you even make it to the finish line? No doubt you would be breathing hard and sweating profusely. Your heart would be bouncing off your chest wall like a trampoline. And it took less than 20 seconds.

For contrast, now imagine walking around the same track for an hour. How would you feel afterwards?

Sure your legs would feel a bit heavy, but that's it. Sweat? Only if it's hot and humid out, but forget about the pounding heart and hard breathing.

What separates the two scenarios is intensity. In the first case you are feeling the effects of pushing your body. In the second case, you're not.

In less than 20 seconds, your body experienced profound changes, something that doesn't come from an hour's worth of walking. What accounts for the difference? One word: Adrenaline, the hormone of intensity.

Sweating, the rapid, bounding pulse, the quickened breathing rate you felt at the end of your run were all signs that adrenaline was ready and eager to burn fat.

Your walk around the track put adrenaline back to sleep.

Exercise intensity is not subjective. It can be measured by not one, but three body gauges. They are:

1. sweating
2. breathing hard and fast
3. having a rapid, bounding pulse

These are three sure physical signs that you are exercising vigorously enough to burn fat. Some patients tell me that after a few minutes of an intense mini-workout, they can almost *taste* their heartbeat. That's intense.

Some say that they feel like kids again.

Catherine T., a psychologist, has the right perspective. "We live in a numb society," she told me. "Adults, unlike children who play hard, hardly ever play hard enough to get their heart rates up, sweat, or breathe hard. Outside of amusement park rides, or being scared momentarily, or sex, it just doesn't happen."

You can change it all around by making exercise a thrilling experience that you look forward to, not a chore.

ADDING INTENSITY

Practically speaking, there are three ways to increase intensity: You do the movements in rapid fashion, or you add force to each movement, or both. Don't just move a leg, kick it out. Don't flail an arm, punch it out like in the martial arts. When you bend, bend all the way.

Move your body with purpose. Get your heart pumping and your lungs burning. Do your three exercises as if you were running the 100-yard dash, not like a leisurely walk around the track.

If you don't need to shower after you exercise, chances are that you still haven't found your intense self yet. How many people do you know who elevate their heart rates voluntarily on a daily basis? Not many.

Then you start the trend. Concentrate your efforts, concentrate your adrenaline.

Concentrate on losing the fat you want to lose.

CHAPTER ELEVEN

MAKING 7 YOUR LUCKY NUMBER

As a child growing up in the rough East New York section of Brooklyn, we played a great game called Seven Minutes in Heaven. The goal was to end up in a bedroom or bathroom, door closed, lights out, with someone of the opposite sex for 7 minutes.

The game had one rule: Don't get caught!

All right, there were two rules: Once 7 minutes passed, your turn was up.

Apparently we weren't the only ones who played the game. Jennifer Connelly, who won the 2002 Oscar for best supporting actress for *A Beautiful Mind*, even starred in a 1985 teen comedy called *Seven Minutes in Heaven*.

Funny. Looking back, how many 5-year-olds can even tell time? Yet, that 7-minute time frame always stuck with me. Whether you played games as a child, or play them now as an adult, I want 7 minutes to be a number that sticks with you, too.

Seven minutes. Four-hundred and twenty seconds.

In less time than it takes to dress to go the gym, you can exercise and slim your most troublesome body area.

WHY 7 MINUTES? IT'S BRAINS OVER BRAWN

In case you're wondering, I didn't just pick 7 minutes because of my fond childhood memories. Like everything else in this program, it's based on sound science. In fact, exercising for longer than 7 minutes gets you diminishing returns, not increased fat loss. The reason: The optimal duration of a spot-reducing workout is determined by brains, not brawn.

It all comes down to this: Does exercise decrease appetite? Or does it make you hungrier than Yogi Bear at a Jellystone Park post-hybernation picnic?

For years, we thought exercise kills our desire to eat. Now, we know differently. Short periods of exercise *don't* increase appetite, but long periods *do!*

It's all because of a brain hormone called neuropeptide Y.

Neuropepetide Y is made in the hypothalamus, a walnut-sized gland embedded deep in your brain. The hypothalamus may be small, but it does big things, like control your sex drive, your sleep patterns, and your mood. Most important of all, it controls your appetite. That's what I call one-stop shopping.

Incidentally, this is the same brain area where antidepressant drugs like Zoloft, Prozac, Paxil, and Celexa do their thing to make us happier.

Neuropeptide Y is your brain's exercise watchdog, protecting and defending you against the possibility, however remote, of exercising yourself to death. While few of us have to worry about something this drastic, leave it to Mother Nature to think of everything.

Neuropepetide Y is a potent appetite stimulator. It goes to work whenever you work out too much.

Immediately following a bout of exercise, neuropeptide Y levels rise, stimulating the hunger center of your brain. The net effect is to make you hungry for a few hours, forcing you to eat more than usual to compensate for any calorie losses from the exercise. This all takes place unconsciously.

Willpower and the best of intentions are no match for this primordial brain mechanism.

DO THE MATH

Two hourly calorie-burning charts will help illustrate how difficult it is to lose weight through traditional exercise. The first chart lists 11 common exercises, with separate columns for men and women. The second chart lists how many calories you burn per hour while working in and around your home.

The values listed are those per hour for a 145-pound woman and a 185-pound man, roughly the weights of the average American woman and man.

The column on the far right shows how many calories an hour are burned per pound of body weight.

■ COMMON EXERCISES

Activity	145-lb Woman	185-lb Man	Calories Burned Per Pound
Cycling	232	296	1.6
Golf	174	222	1.2
Ping Pong	362	462	2.5
Rowing	725	925	5.0
Running	536	684	3.7
Skating	304	388	2.1
Skiing	754	962	5.2
Swimming	580	740	4.0
Tennis	406	518	2.8
Walking	203	259	1.4

Calculating the number of calories burned at your body weight is simple. Just multiply your body weight by the number in the far right column of the activity you chose.

For example, suppose you are a 150-pound woman who wants to start walking. First, though, you want to know how many calories you will burn per hour. Find the walking heading on the left side of the chart, then go to the far right column in the "calories burned per pound."

The number is 1.4, or one and four-tenths calories burned each hour for each pound of body weight. Do the math, 150 x 1.4=210 calories.

So if you walk for an hour at moderate pace you will burn 210 calories.

If you walk for half an hour, you use up 105 calories. If you walk for 15 minutes that number shrinks to 52.5 calories.

Patients often ask me why house or office work doesn't help them lose weight. I've prepared a second chart listing how many calories are burned per hour performing various house and office activities. Again, the values are for a typical 145-pound woman and 185-pound man.

■ DAILY CHORES AND ACTIVITIES

	145-lb Woman	185-lb Man	Calories Burned Per Pound
Cooking	116	148	0.8
Gardening	333	425	2.3
Housecleaning	290	370	2.0
Ironing	145	185	1.0
Knitting	101	129	0.7
Laundry	145	185	1.0
Piano playing	159	203	1.1
Sewing	101	129	0.7
Typing	130	166	0.9
Writing	101	129	0.7

Do you realize that walking and playing piano burn about the same number of calories?

This shows two things. First, piano playing is better for you than you thought. Billy Joel and Elton John have it right!

Second, it shows how inefficient walking is for weight loss.

You could watch Billy and Elton pound the keys at New York's Madison Square Garden one night, then—at a rate of 5 miles per hour—walk to Philadelphia, catch them again at the First Union Center 17 hours later, and still lose only 1 pound!

And did you notice that doing laundry burns nearly as many calories as golf? By the way, which of these gets your heart rate up? Neither one.

The few exercises that do get your heart rate up aren't done by most people: running and rowing. Imagine doing either for an hour.

Let's get real once more.

To lose 1 pound of body weight via exercise or while working around the house or office, you need to expend 3,500 calories. From these two charts, it's quite easy to figure how long it would take to burn 3,500 calories and then actually do it. Simply divide 3,500 by the number of calories you burn per hour.

For instance, a 145-pound woman burning 232 calories per hour cycling would need 15 hours just to burn off one pound! It would take a 175-pound woman almost 4 hours to row a pound away!

THE 7-MINUTE SOLUTION

What do all these number really mean?

It's clear that you burn most of your calories when you aren't exercising. And the 7-Minute Miracle Workout is attuned to this fact. Our 7-minute session sets the tone for increased fat-burning for hours later.

I hope that gives you a better perspective on exercise. It should begin to be clear now why, when you got on the scale after weeks of walking or cycling, you weighed exactly the same as before you started.

That's because neuropeptide Y was keeping tabs on the extra calories you were burning, without you being aware, and making sure that you ate the exact amount of food necessary to offset the amount of calories you burned.

The conclusion to reach from all of this is that when it comes to weight loss from exercise, it's not about how much exercise you do, or how many calories you burn.

It's more about coming to grips with some pretty strong brain chemicals stacked against weight loss.

Then how long can you exercise before awaking neuropeptide Y? By now, you shouldn't need a slew of psychic friends to predict the correct answer: It's 7 minutes! Seven minutes of continuous, vigorous exercise is the threshold that will keep neuropeptide Y at bay. Anything more stimulates your appetite and works against spot reducing.

And as powerful as it is, neuropeptide Y doesn't act alone. Its partner in crime is a set of brain chemical called endorphins.

BETTER THAN SEX?

Endorphins are responsible for the so-called "runners' high." This is the mystical, fleeting, intensely positive feeling that can overwhelm your whole body during and shortly after rigorous exercise.

Arnold Schwarzenegger, back in his Mr. Olympia days, once wrote that the "pump"—the weight-lifter's high that hits you when your muscles are engorged with blood following a hard workout—is better than sex.

Having experienced both, I disagree. Sex is definitely better.

But Arnold showed great insight making the comparison because endorphins not only play a role in feeling good, but in female and male orgasms, too. Their love connection aside, endorphins are ultra-powerful appetite enhancers.

Like neuropeptide Y, exercise gets endorphins going. The more you exercise, the more endorphins your brain makes, and the more food they compel you to eat. So exactly how long can you exercise vigorously before your brain unleashes endorphins on your appetite?

I'll make it easy for you. Pick an odd number between 6 and 8.

Did you say 7? That's correct! You don't need a Las Vegas croupier to let you know that your lucky exercise number is 7.

Now you understand that we aren't doing you a favor by limiting your spot workout to 7 minutes. We're just conforming to normal human physiology.

Seven minutes is the right time. It's long enough to allow adrenaline to activate your weight-loss genes and at the same time it's short enough to not arouse your endorphins and neuropeptide Y and increase your appetite.

Keep in mind, though, that what you skimp on in time, you more than make up for with intensity. Few of you will be able to do a full 7-minute workout initially. Do the best you can and with each session, try to prolong the routine even more.

In a theoretical sense, you never will attain the perfect 7-Minute Miracle Workout. Nor would you want to. You never want a ceiling, or a limiting factor on what you can accomplish.

Once you're able to go the full 7 minutes, a case can be made that you could have done the movements with more intensity, or that perhaps the next time out, you could put more oomph! into each movement or go that much faster.

That's entirely up to you.

If you're ready to spend the next 7 minutes burning fat exactly where you want to by doing a quick, heart-pounding, blood-pumping and fat gene-activating routine, then let's get to it.

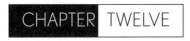

CHAPTER TWELVE

THE 7-MINUTE MIRACLE WORKOUT

Odds are, you've tried exercising before. Probably many different times, many different ways. But I'm pretty sure about one thing: You've never tried exercising the 7-Minute Miracle way.

So before we get to the actual exercises, let me take you through a typical workout.

First of all: Don't answer the doorbell! You've committed to spending your 7 minutes a day, and those 7 minutes have to be in one fell swoop. Don't try to do these in 2-minute bursts between phone calls or helping your daughter with her homework! Make sure you pick a time and place where you won't be disturbed or distracted. Believe me, you'll need all the concentration you can get while you're working your 7-Minute Miracle!

The steps in the exercises are labeled, making it easy to follow along with the models in the photos. Most have a starting, middle, and ending position, as noted. Go over them in your mind before you start.

The 7-Minute Miracle Workout Q&A

Three questions about The 7-Minute Miracle's exercise plan seem to pop up most often. They are:

QUESTION 1: I already exercise. How do I integrate The 7-Minute Miracle Workout into my regular routine?

First off, I salute any of you who exercise regularly. No matter what type of exercise you do, don't stop! You know how strongly I feel about exercise. Living is moving, moving is living.

But whether you jog, run the treadmill, play basketball, or swim, let me offer one guideline: Separate your normal routine from your 7-Minute Miracle Workout by at least 3 hours. And longer is even better.

In other words, don't tag 7 minutes of spot-reducing exercise onto your regular workout. Traditional exercise, as I've discussed, dilutes your spot fat-burning capabilities because there simply isn't enough adrenaline to go around.

Once your regular routine is over, your body is spent, because it's used up some of its stores of potential spot-reducing enzymes and hormones.

To get out of this depleted state, your body needs at least 3 hours of rest, depending on the individual. Think of this interval as your body re-charging its own weight-loss batteries.

Practically speaking, this isn't such a big deal. Those of you who exercise in the morning can do the spot-reducing routine at night. Those of you who work out at night can spot themselves 7 in the morning.

Once you've chosen which hot spot you want to work on first, go to that section—Belly, Butt, Thighs, Hips, or Arms—and begin with exercise #1, starting position.

Follow the movement along with the model through the middle position onto the ending position in one motion. Repeat this pattern over again without counting. While you move, focus on your body in motion, almost like yoga, without assigning a number to each movement.

QUESTION 2: How often should I exercise?

When it comes to workout frequency, more is better. How many 7-minute sessions per week burn the most fat as quickly as possible? The short answer is 7!

I suggest that for optimum results, you do The 7-Minute Miracle Workout daily. So what's the fewest weekly workouts you can get away with and still achieve results? Four times a week seems to be the minimum that need to be done for fat cell activation to take place. Anything less, and your weight-loss genes go back to sleep. Three times a week is sufficent if you're working exercises on alternate days (see page 85).

Also, take care not to go more than 2 days between workouts. The time off makes your genes "rusty."

QUESTION 3: How long before I see results?

Each of you has an inherent metabolic switch inside that determines your rate of weight loss. However, since we're measuring body part sizes not body part weights, it takes days, not weeks, before most of you can measure your progress either objectively with the pinch test or looser clothes, or subjectively by looking in the mirror with or without your clothes!

Keep in mind that the program begins working the moment you finish your 7-minute workout. Yet because there are millions of fat cells at each hot spot, it takes a few days' time to get enough of them to dump out their fat, so that you can feel and see the difference.

A word about breathing: It's important to remember to breathe while you move through these exercises. Holding your breath will only exhaust you sooner, and will keep you from getting the most out of each exercise. Breathe in through your nose at the beginning of each movement, and exhale through your lips on exertion (the hard parts!).

At some point, fatigue will set in and you'll experience the annoying burning sensation of muscle fatigue in the hot spot you're working on.

This natural phenomenon is caused by the build-up of the waste product lactic acid in your muscles. It is your body's defense against overuse.

Don't try to override it. Don't fight through it. Forget the dumb and discredited saying, "No pain, no gain." And let me say here, just to be clear: Intensity is *not* measured in pain. It's measured in effort. There's a big difference.

Immediately move on to the starting position of exercise #2 and follow along with the model to the ending position until you feel the lactic acid build up once more.

At this point, move on to the first position of exercise #3 and proceed to do as much as you can, going from starting to ending position and back again, until you tire once more. Then return to the starting position of exercise #1 and repeat the cycle again until your 7 minutes are up.

Try to give each movement equal billing in terms of time. If you tend to favor one movement over the other two, that's okay, as long as you spend at least some time with your least favorite exercise.

Remember, no one exercise is more important than the others. In this case, it takes three to tango! And these exercises should be a dance. Do them to music, or make your own music. As you move in one continuous loop, you create your own internal rhythm.

It's electric! Before long, you will actually feel your insides dancing, a whole different feeling than you get from mere exercise.

Though these exercises look easy on paper, they are not paper exercises. They are so challenging that few if any of you will be able to last 7 minutes the first few times out. Consider yourself fit (and lucky!) if you last more than 2 or 3 minutes.

Yet with each routine that you do, your muscles get smarter. It's as if they can do the exercises by themselves, with you in command, of course.

What I have just described is the official 7-Minute Miracle Workout. It's valid for all five hot spots.

When you do yours, remember:

• No sets, no reps.

- Keep moving fluidly and ignore the exercise police.
- Don't count.
- Listen to your body. It's telling you to make it intense.

THE TWO-FOR-ONE SPECIAL

I know what many of you are thinking: What if I have more than one hot spot I want to lose? Is there any way to hit more than one at a time?

The answer, you'll be glad to hear, is, yes. Over time, you can lose weight from other areas besides the targeted hot spot that you initially choose. Certain areas like the thighs and hips just seem to go together like good tongue-and-groove construction. Shrink one and you can often shrink the other, without doing the specific exercises for the second site. Because they share blood vessels, every 7-Minute Miracle thigh workout, for example, sends fat-burning adrenaline over to trim your hips and vice-versa.

For those of you who want to shrink two hot spots at the same time that aren't anatomically related, like the arms and tush, we use a simple, alternate-day strategy.

Do your 7-minute workout for arms one day and then next day work on your tush. Repeat this pattern on alternating days, always following up, of course, with the 40-minute pause and The 7-Minute Miracle meal. Use this alternate-day strategy to shrink the two hot spots of your choice.

Sorry, Charlie: What you can't do is add the 7 minutes of one body site to the 7 minutes of another site for a 14-minute workout, nor can you do a 35-minute workout and get at all the areas!

Remember, the magic number is 7. Any workout longer than 7 minutes will dilute your adrenaline too much and increase your appetite.

THE 7-MINUTE BUTT WORKOUT

■ BENT KNEE LIFTS

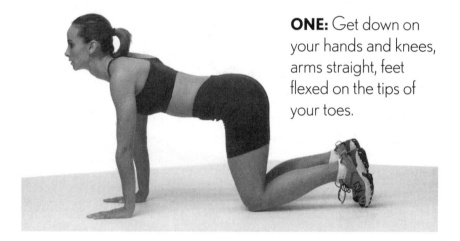

ONE: Get down on your hands and knees, arms straight, feet flexed on the tips of your toes.

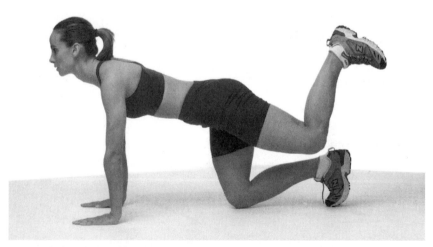

TWO: Lift left leg back and up, keeping your knee bent, and your back flat.

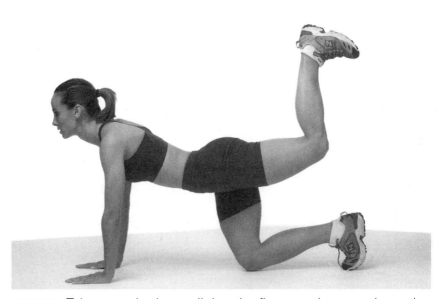

THREE: Take your thigh parallel to the floor, pushing up through your heel, foot flexed. Repeat to exhaustion, then switch legs.

■ MAKE IT INTENSE!

Squeeze the muscles surrounding your knee as you push up through your heel.

THE WRONG WAY

Don't arch your back or hyper-extend your leg beyond parallel to the floor.

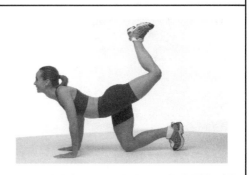

THE 7-MINUTE BUTT WORKOUT

■ PRONE LEG LIFTS

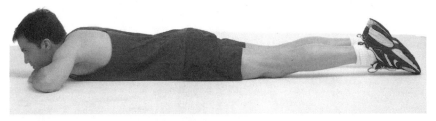

ONE: Lie on the floor face down, arms crossed in front of you, your chin resting on your hands.

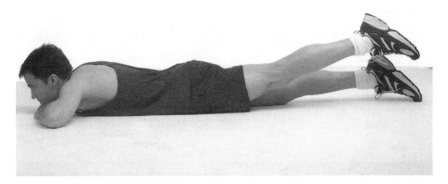

TWO: Slowly lift left leg just a few inches off the floor, keeping your hips on the floor.

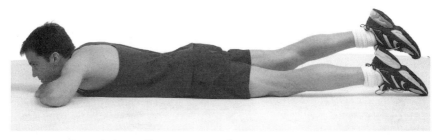

THREE: Switch legs. Repeat to exhaustion.

■ MAKE IT INTENSE!

This exercise is built for speed: Switch quickly from right leg to left leg, as if you were swimming.

THE WRONG WAY

Don't hyper-extend your leg or allow your hips to come up off the floor.

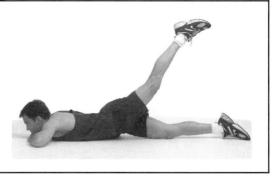

THE 7-MINUTE BUTT WORKOUT

■ FANNY LIFTS

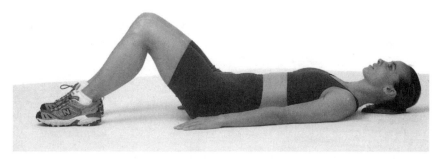

ONE: Lie on your back, knees bent, with your feet flat on the floor. Your arms are at your sides.

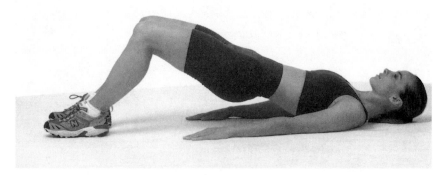

TWO: Raise your hips and fanny as high off the floor as you can, keeping your upper back flat on the floor. Squeeze your fanny muscles, and relax, slowly returning to starting position.

■ MAKE IT INTENSE!
Push your feet hard down into the floor as you raise your fanny.

THE 7-MINUTE HIPS WORKOUT

■ SIDE LIFTS

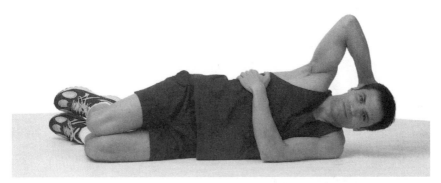

ONE: Lie on your left side, legs together, knees bent. Keep your knees in line with your hips and shoulders. You're leaning on your left arm, your right arm is behind your head.

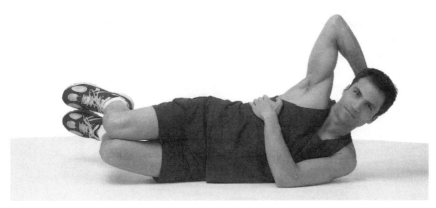

TWO: Lift both thighs and knees together, and lift your torso at the same time. Release and return to starting position.

■ MAKE IT INTENSE!
This exercise is intense enough, believe me!

THE 7-MINUTE HIPS WORKOUT

■ HIP EXTENSIONS

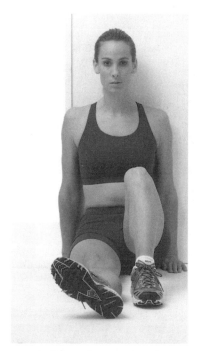

ONE: Sit with your back against the wall, left knee bent, right leg straight out in front of you, foot turned out.

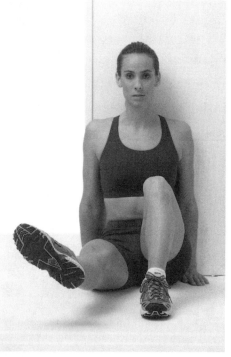

TWO: Lift right leg up 3 to 4 inches off the floor.

THREE: Gently rotate your right leg out to the side, feeling the pull in your hips, and return to starting position. Repeat to exhaustion, then switch legs.

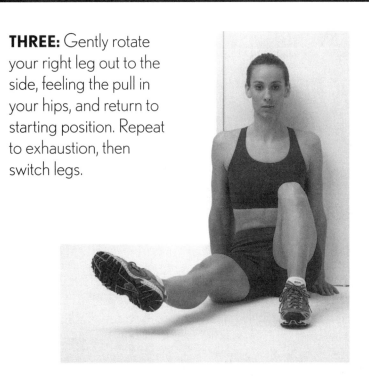

THE WRONG WAY

Keep your hips close to the wall, don't shift your hip to lift your leg higher than 4 inches.

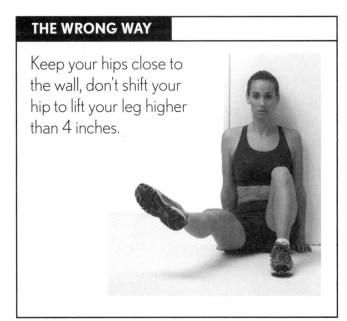

THE 7-MINUTE HIPS WORKOUT

■ SIDE CIRCLES

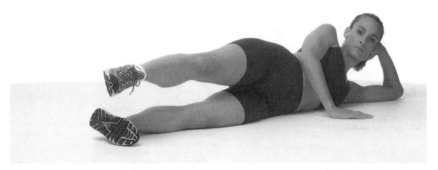

ONE: Lie on your left side with your head propped up on your left hand, your left arm across the front of you, hand flat on the floor. Your legs are straight, knees together, and feet flexed.

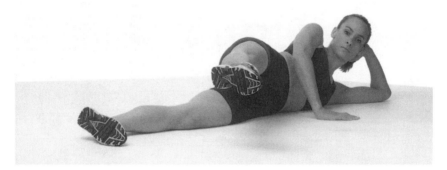

TWO: Raise your top (right) leg slightly and begin to bring it forward.

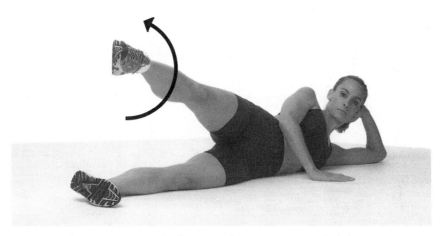

THREE: Rotate your right leg up, then over your left leg.

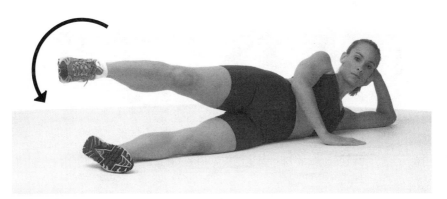

FOUR: Continue moving your leg slightly behind you, then return to starting position, completing a circle in the air. Repeat to exhaustion, then switch legs.

■ MAKE IT INTENSE!

These can be done slowly, but for a really intense experience, make tight, rapid circles with your active leg.

THE 7-MINUTE THIGHS WORKOUT

■ THE GENIE

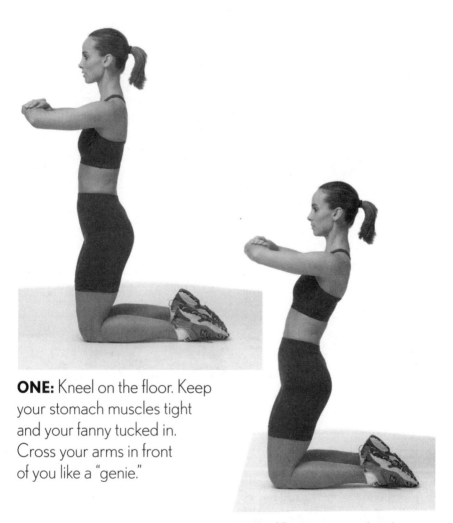

ONE: Kneel on the floor. Keep your stomach muscles tight and your fanny tucked in. Cross your arms in front of you like a "genie."

TWO: Keeping your back straight, lean back as far as you can.

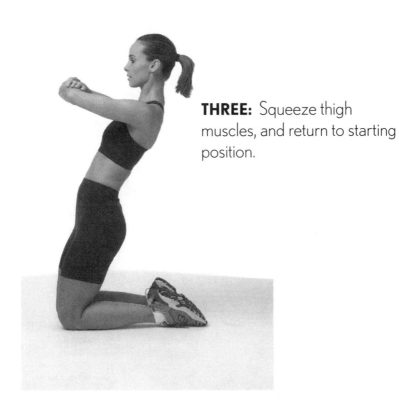

THREE: Squeeze thigh muscles, and return to starting position.

■ MAKE IT INTENSE!

This one's intense enough! Whew!

THE 7-MINUTE THIGHS WORKOUT

■ SUMO SQUATS

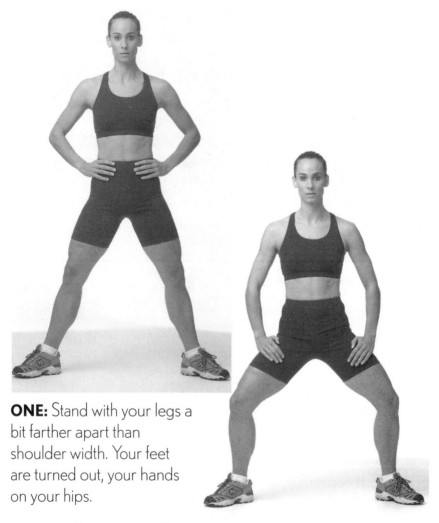

ONE: Stand with your legs a bit farther apart than shoulder width. Your feet are turned out, your hands on your hips.

TWO: Keeping your back straight, and your eyes looking straight ahead of you (not up) begin to lower your fanny to the floor. Slide your hands down to rest on your thighs for balance.

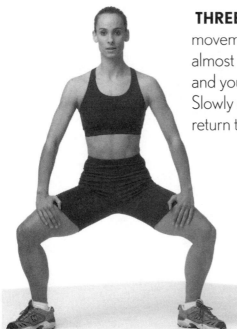

THREE: Continue squatting movement until your thighs are almost at right angles to the floor, and you feel the pull in your thighs. Slowly reverse the movement and return to starting position.

■ MAKE IT INTENSE!

Remember to keep your fanny tucked in and your stomach muscles tight.

THE WRONG WAY

Don't squat so far that your thighs are parallel to the floor.

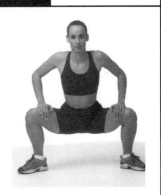

THE 7-MINUTE THIGHS WORKOUT

■ SIDE LEG RAISES

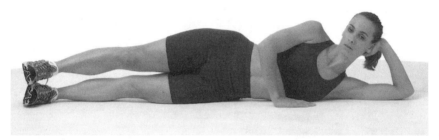

ONE: Lie on your left side with your head propped up on your left hand, your right arm crossed in front of you, hand flat on the floor. Your legs are straight, knees together.

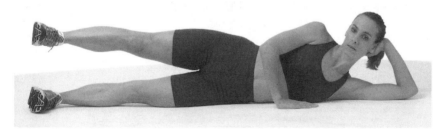

TWO: Slowly raise your top (right) leg to just above your hips.

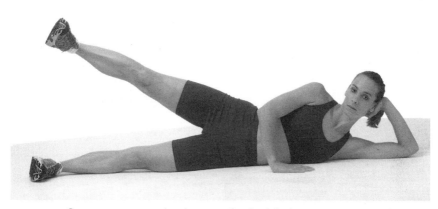

THREE: Squeeze your thigh muscle, hold, then return to starting position. Repeat to exhaustion, then switch legs.

■ MAKE IT INTENSE!

Push your opposite hip hard into the floor as you raise your leg.

THE WRONG WAY

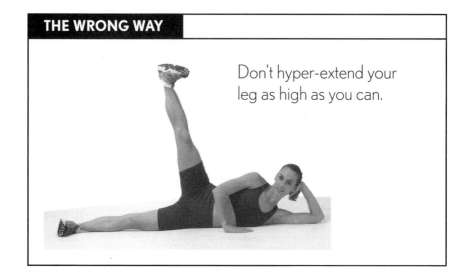

Don't hyper-extend your leg as high as you can.

THE 7-MINUTE ARMS WORKOUT

■ KICKBACKS

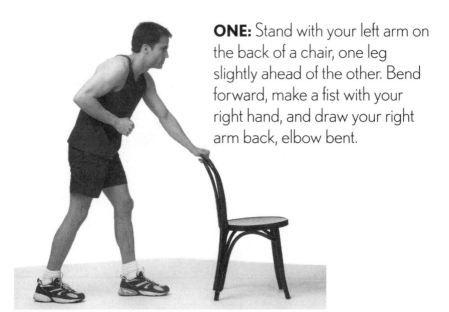

ONE: Stand with your left arm on the back of a chair, one leg slightly ahead of the other. Bend forward, make a fist with your right hand, and draw your right arm back, elbow bent.

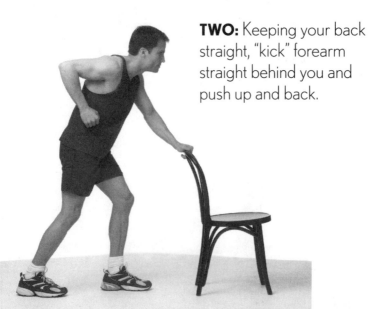

TWO: Keeping your back straight, "kick" forearm straight behind you and push up and back.

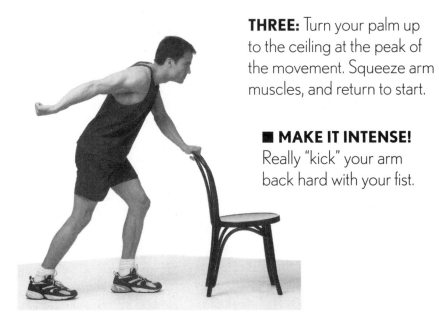

THREE: Turn your palm up to the ceiling at the peak of the movement. Squeeze arm muscles, and return to start.

■ MAKE IT INTENSE!
Really "kick" your arm back hard with your fist.

THE WRONG WAY

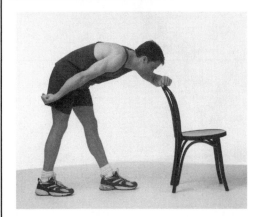

Don't bend at the waist or slump over. Try to keep your back at a 45-degree angle.

THE 7-MINUTE ARMS WORKOUT

■ ARM WALL PRESS

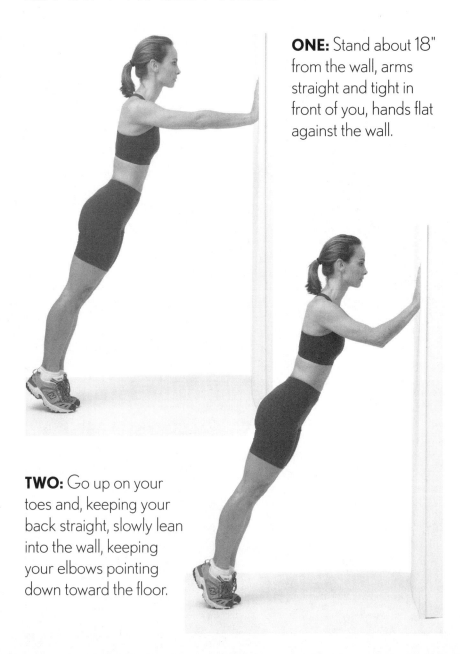

ONE: Stand about 18" from the wall, arms straight and tight in front of you, hands flat against the wall.

TWO: Go up on your toes and, keeping your back straight, slowly lean into the wall, keeping your elbows pointing down toward the floor.

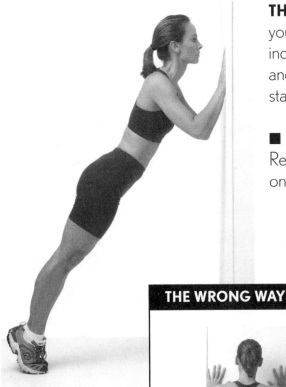

THREE: Stop when your head is about 2 inches from the wall, and push back out to starting position.

■ **MAKE IT INTENSE!** Remember to stay high on your toes.

THE WRONG WAY

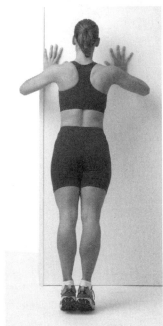

Don't flex your elbows out to the side.

THE 7-MINUTE ARMS WORKOUT

■ KARATE THRUSTS

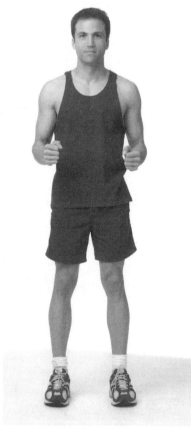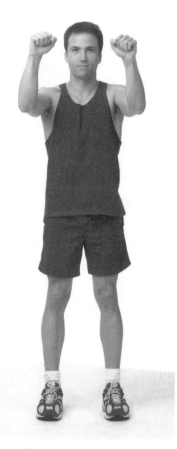

ONE: Stand with your legs shoulder-width apart. Bring your forearms up, elbows at your sides, and make a fist with both hands.

TWO: Raise your arms up halfway, turning your fists palm-out as you do so.

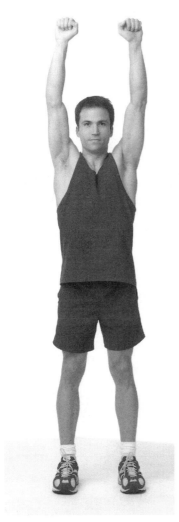

THE WRONG WAY

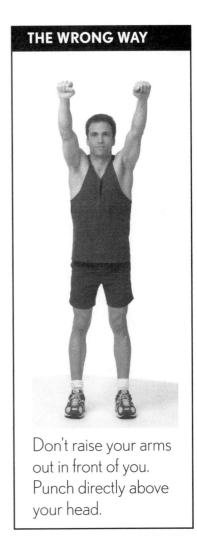

Don't raise your arms out in front of you. Punch directly above your head.

THREE: Raise your arms up above your head, punching the air with your fists. Quickly bring your arms back down to the starting position.

■ MAKE IT INTENSE!
Use forceful thrusts when moving your arms both up and down.

THE 7-MINUTE BELLY WORKOUT

■ BOXER LIFTS

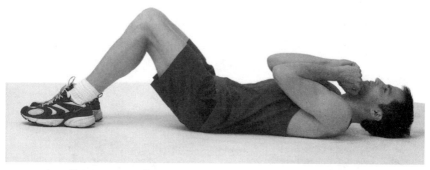

ONE: Lie flat on your back, with your knees bent. Your arms and wrists are bent in a "boxer" stance.

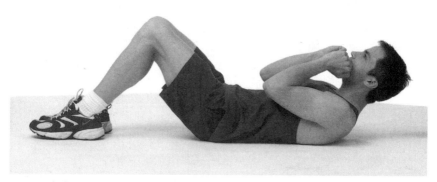

TWO: Lift your top torso 2 inches off the floor.

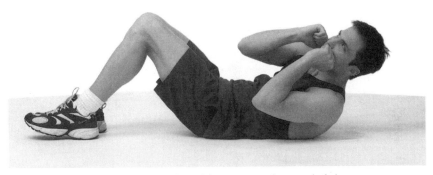

THREE: Bend your right shoulder toward your left knee.

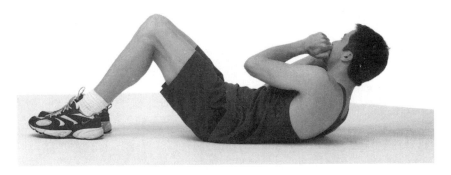

FOUR: Then turn your left shoulder toward your right knee. Return to the starting position and repeat to exhaustion.

■ MAKE IT INTENSE!

Really twist your torso and "torque" your shoulder toward the opposing knee.

THE 7-MINUTE BELLY WORKOUT

■ BICYCLES

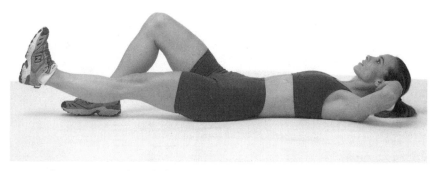

ONE: Lie on your back, hands behind your head, with your elbows flat.

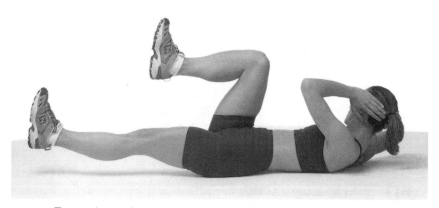

TWO: Extend one leg out straight and tight, your foot flexed. The other leg is bent toward your chest.

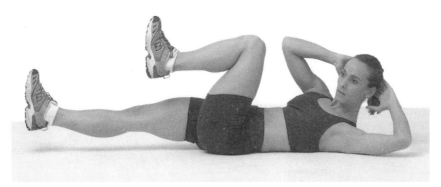

THREE: While alternating legs, like riding a bicycle, lift up and twist your upper body right to meet your left knee, then left to meet your right knee. Continue to exhaustion.

■ MAKE IT INTENSE!

This exercise is custom-made for speed. Keep those legs pumping!

THE WRONG WAY

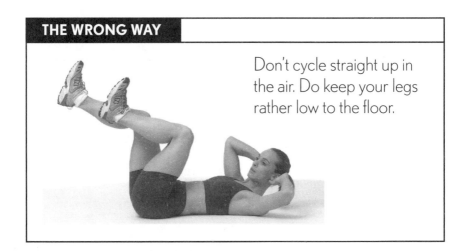

Don't cycle straight up in the air. Do keep your legs rather low to the floor.

THE 7-MINUTE BELLY WORKOUT

■ PUNCHES

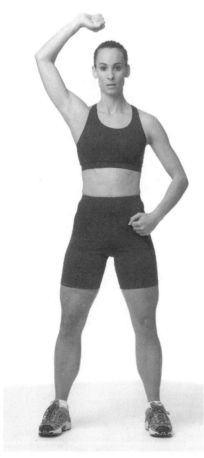 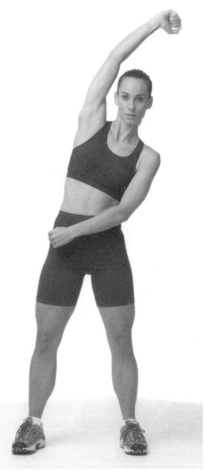

ONE: Assume a wide stance, keeping legs and buttocks tight. Make a fist with both hands.

TWO: With your right arm over your head, punch to the left, while punching to the right with your left arm across your abdomen.

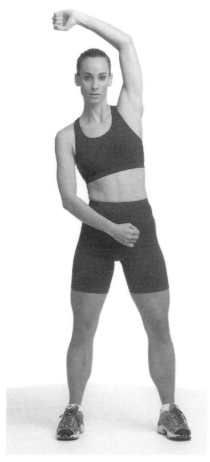

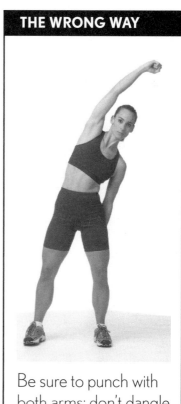

THE WRONG WAY

Be sure to punch with both arms; don't dangle your lower arm.

THREE: Continue to exhaustion, then switch arms.

MAKE IT INTENSE: Be sure to thrust your lower arm forcefully across your body, almost pulling your body in two different directions as you punch your opposite arm above you.

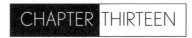

CHAPTER THIRTEEN

PAUSE FOR THE CAUSE: NO FOOD FOR 40

Sometimes you have to pause to keep on going. This is one of those times.

Once you finish your 7 minutes of fat-busting exercises, there's only one thing to do, or better yet, *not* to do: Don't eat for 40 minutes.

While your spot-reducing workout starts the ball rolling, most of your fat-burning occurs after you finish exercising. To continue the fat-burning at your belly, butt, thighs, hips, or arms that began 7 minutes ago, you need a 40-minute timeout from food.

Please, don't make me beg. Please, no food for 40 minutes.

Hey, that would make a great slogan: No food for 40!

DON'T GUM UP YOUR FAT-BURNING FURNACE

Think of the 40-minute pause as a no-fly zone over your stomach. But when I say no food I mean, no food: nada, zilch, niente, zero. And no drinks either, except for water.

Eating or drinking anything but water right after exercise is a huge mistake, because it brings fat-burning to a halt. Let me explain why.

Your stomach and your fat cells are connected. No, not connected like on *The Sopranos*, but connected physically. Certain hormones and nerve endings connect your digestive system to your fat cells. The presence of food in the stomach stretches the stomach wall, sending a signal to the rest of the body—including your fat cells—that more blood is needed in the area to aid with digestion.

This immediately diverts precious blood and adrenaline away from your belly, butt, thighs, hips, and arms to your stomach, which slows fat-burning down like a tortoise jogging in wet concrete.

The news gets even worse if you eat fat in the first 40 minutes immediately after exercise.

Fatty foods like fries, chips, and cheese stimulate your pancreas to secrete its own brand of fat-digesting lipase into the stomach and blood. At the same time, your fat cells are ordered to not only stop all fat-burning, but to reverse the fat-burning process.

The result: New fat gets deposited in your fat cells, not burned! This means that fat eaten immediately following exercise causes weight gain, not weight loss. Keep in mind that many energy and protein bars contain fat in varying amounts, so take special care to avoid them.

No food in the stomach for 40 minutes prevents the detour of adrenaline and lipase away from where they are needed most, your five hot spots. And almost all drinks, except water, contain the same protein, carbohydrates, and fats found in solid food. That's why you should pass on juices, sodas, protein, and even energizing and recovery drinks.

Also, avoid caffeinated drinks because they are natural diuretics, depleting us of water and electrolytes—key minerals such as potassium, calcium, and magnesium that carry electrical charges that help regulate hydration and muscle movement. After we exercise we want to conserve water and electrolytes, not lose them.

WATER: LIQUID MAGIC

The English author D.H. Lawrence said that water is two parts hydrogen, one part oxygen, and one part magic.

During your 40-minute pause, water can work magic for you. Increasing your water intake during the 40-minute pause makes up for the water you used while exercising and sweating.

Plus, when you burn fat, water is liberated from fat cells and eventually gets excreted in your urine. When you drink water, you replace the water that you lose in this fashion.

I know that recovery drinks are real hot now, but take my advice: Water is much cooler. Recovery drinks contain specific combinations of carbohydrates, protein, and fat. They are designed to help your muscles recover from an arduous muscle-burning workout.

They may work wonders for your muscles, but recovery drinks are not kind to your fat cells. In the end, they do the same thing that solid food does: divert blood from your fat cells to your stomach.

You don't want that to happen, do you?

In any event, the 40-minute no-eating break passes quickly. Think of it as a temporary bridge linking your 7-minute, spot-reducing workout to the spot meal that follows. But don't just wait around for that bonsai plant to grow. Do something!

Depending on when you exercise, there is plenty for you to do, like shower, shave, read, or even make love. The latter comes highly recommended because sexual hormones that make you hornier than a caged rabbit flow vigorously right after your 7-Minute Miracle Workout.

Weightlifters and bodybuilders have long claimed that making love right after a tough training session is best. Find out for yourself.

To recap, do anything you like over the 40-minute pause, except eat. After all, the tastiest part of the Genetic Body Sculpting Plan is yet to come: The 7-Minute Miracle Meal.

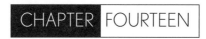

CHAPTER FOURTEEN

FOOD POWER:
EAT YOUR HOT SPOTS AWAY

Now we come to the best part. This is where you actually eat yourself thin.

The 7-Minute Miracle Workout and the 40-minute, no-eating pause have boosted your metabolism and your fat-burning capabilities. In other words, the table is set and it's time to eat.

You have about a 6-hour window of opportunity for continued fat-burning, so what you put on your plate now is important. Certain foods prod your genes to continue fat-burning, while others turn the genes off, guaranteeing that fat-burning grinds to a halt.

The 7-Minute Miracle Meal loads up on gene-activating foods and avoids those that send your genes to snoozeville. It works only when it follows The 7-Minute Miracle Workout. As Sinatra sang about love and marriage: you can't have one without the other.

The fat-burning process begun by your workout is not complete without the spot meal, while the spot meal has no ability to foster fat burning unless it's preceded by the exercise. The 7-Minute Miracle Meal is the third and final part of The 7-Minute Miracle Genetic Body Sculpting Plan.

And best of all, one 7-Minute Miracle Meal Plan covers all of your body's hot spots.

THE MEAL THAT MATTERS MOST

Many of you may not realize that the food you eat after you exercise can make or break your weight-loss fortunes. For starters, eating high-fat foods after you work out can negate the amount of calories you burned, making your workout a washout.

And it gets worse: Eating just a single high-fat meal after intense exercise can cancel your workout benefits for up to two days. The flip side of this is the good news: A single 7-Minute Miracle Meal can make all the difference.

And here's even better news: You'll never have to go on a diet again.

Diets. Like your last lover, you've tried them, fallen hopelessly in love, hated them, then thrown them out forever—only to take them back the next day.

Whether you have a small nib of extra fat on your thighs or un-wanted padding on your hips, at some point you probably asked the same question that people ask me every day: "What should I eat?"

There is one simple truth about diets. Whether, it's low-carbohy-drate, high-protein, or low-fat, no animal on earth likes to voluntarily cut their food intake, especially us. Stephanie L., a writer from Rock-land County, New York, put it best: "I once went on a diet for four-teen days, and all I lost were two weeks."

With the 7-Minute Miracle Meal, you only have to watch what you eat after you exercise. The rest of the day is yours.

As you now know, your body has the ability to stay at a high level of fat-burning for about 6 hours after you exercise, courtesy of your weight-control genes. That's why the post-exercise period interests us most. What you eat in the period before you exercise, when your fat cells are back to their resting state, doesn't matter as much.

Now, if you're one of those who insist that you must diet to succeed, consider yourselves on a once-a-day diet.

Are you happy now?

But you won't be left out to dry the rest of the day.

We'll show you how to fine-tune your food intake for your other meals so that if you love chocolate or cookies, you can indulge and still do well. If you are salt of the earth and crave salty foods, you can have your daily fix and still trim your thighs or belly.

GENE-FRIENDLY FOODS

Foods are either gene-friendly or they aren't. Either they stimulate your fat cells to burn fat or they don't. To figure out which food does what, scientists used the same abdominal clamp technique I relied on to develop The 7-Minute Miracle Workout.

Researchers would continuously put ingredients made of carbohydrates, protein, fats, and fiber into one end of the catheter and wait to see how much messenger RNA (mRNA) came out of the other end. mRNA, as you'll recall, is a substance made by your genes inside fat cells, and the amount that comes out of the tube tells us whether the foods in question activated the fat cells.

Big jumps in mRNA mean gene activation and potential fat-burning. No spike in mRNA signifies that the genes are inactive and sleeping. From the research, a definitive fat cell-activating formula emerged that forms the basis for The 7-Minute Miracle Meal.

Since we know what your body wants to eat and we focus on one single meal, this has to be the easiest eating plan ever. To eliminate any chance of error, we have precise menu plans for you, which give brand names and exact portion sizes, so that you can give your own expert answer to the question, "What should I eat?"

The spot meal may be eaten as breakfast, lunch, or dinner, depending on when you exercise. Most people exercise in the morning or evening, so breakfast or dinner will be your spot meal.

For those of you who work out over your lunch break at work, The 7-Minute Miracle Workout can easily be finished with 53 minutes to spare in your lunch hour! Also, a lot of new moms tell me that they get some time for themselves at around noon, when a new baby, up all night, finally falls asleep. For all of you afternoon enthusiasts, we have a great spot lunch.

The real beauty of The 7-Minute Miracle Meal is that it not only does great things for your body, it works wonders for your head, too. Oftentimes, patients put me in the role of a priest taking confession. They view their eating travails as the battle between good and evil.

If someone's able to watch their food intake closely and lose weight, they are quick to say, not that they were successful, but they were good. Should they stray, they're not unsuccessful, they're bad.

Sometimes they come into my office looking like condemned prisoners, head down, waiting for their punishment, perhaps to be burned at the stake of dieting heresy.

I remind them that I'm a doctor, not the grand inquisitor. I remind them that when it comes to losing weight, saints turn into sinners and sinners into saints ten to twenty times a day.

The 7-Minute Miracle Meal empowers you to forget about being good or bad, and concentrate on giving your body what it wants and needs once a day.

Patients tell me that when they wake up in the morning, they are in an instant good mood, knowing that the pressure of dieting is off. They only have to concentrate on one meal per day. Some look at it as a release from that horrible feeling of always having to be on guard against their own refrigerators.

For others, the 7-Minute Miracle Meal is a refuge. The human mind craves order. Your body craves balance. The spot meal is composed of a precise qualitative and quantitative eating formula that is easy on your body and leaves nothing to chance.

However, should you not make the greatest food choices at other times during the day, you can still fall back on your 7 minutes of spot-reducing exercise and the spot meal that follows, knowing you haven't blown it completely.

You do your part, and your body will do all it can to help you, especially since you won't be starving it, or shoving tons of slimy fats and heavy-duty protein into it.

The first part of the unspoken pact between you and your body is that your 7-minute spot reducing workout *decreases* your appetite, making it much easier to concentrate on the one spot meal.

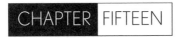

A FORMULA
FOR SUCCESS

When it comes to losing weight, the High-Low game is the biggest con this side of Three-Card Monte. Whether you bet on high carbohydrates, or low carbohydrates; high protein, or low protein; high fat, or low fat, you're bound to lose. It's what's known in Brooklyn as a sucker's bet.

I know a lot of my patients have played the game, and paid the price.

In just one morning recently, patient after patient told me about their latest fad diet. These are all smart people. They just got bad information.

Mary P., a 45-year-old town supervisor, laments that she's addicted to carbs. "They make me sluggish, especially in midafternoon," she said.

A few minutes later, Francine G., an attorney and mother of two who recently began training for the New York Marathon, told me carbs aren't the problem, they're the solution.

"I can't live without carbs. I need them for energy. Besides, nearly all world-class marathoners load up on pasta and bread before they compete," she said.

Next up was Sue M., a 39-year-old registered nurse, who told me how she just went to the bookstore and "discovered" the Pritikin plan. I told her that program was older than my Partridge Family records.

"Mmm, it's new to me," she said, sheepishly.

That same morning, I had other patients tell me they were eating according to their blood type or matching their food intake by color, like wallpaper. Others were trying to find their Zone or were lost in Hollywood.

When it comes to weight loss, there's only one expert you should listen to about food. And that's your body. The 7-Minute Miracle Meal is based on a formula derived by examining the direct effects of carbohydrates, fats, and protein on your fat cells.

Talk about listening to your body. You can't make a more intimate connection between what you eat and losing weight than that.

So what is the magic formula? Well, it's actually more science than magic. But what can happen to your body if you follow this formula truly is magical: carbohydrates, 50 percent; fat, 30 percent; protein, 20 percent; plus fiber.

In other words, one-half of each 7-Minute Miracle Meal is made up of delicious carbohydrates, fat makes up about one-third, and protein one-fifth.

Notice that no quantity of fiber is given. Though fiber has been shown to help burn fat, the precise amount or even the type of fiber which works best hasn't been worked out yet.

In any event, every 7-Minute Miracle Meal contains ample fiber.

Remember, I don't make the rules. Your body does. The ingredients of The 7-Minute Miracle Meal were drawn from direct human research. That's why high protein, high fat, or high *anything* is out.

A balanced, healthy meal is in, one that can do something that no other way of eating can: help burn fat in the post-exercise period.

To those of you who prefer a different way of eating, be my guest! You have two other meals each day where you can do your own thing.

Let's take a brief look at how we plug protein, fat, carbohydrates, and fiber into each 7-Minute Miracle Meal, beginning with the least utilized macronutrient, protein.

PROTEIN: GOING AGAINST THE GRAIN

If you've gotten caught up in the recent high-protein mania, you know that The 7-Minute Miracle Meal goes against the grain of what's out there now. Personally, I believe the high-protein fad peaked about 5 minutes ago.

The word protein comes from the Greek word *proteus,* for primary. But in The 7-Minute Miracle Meal, protein is not a primary player.

That's because the dietary protein found in meat, eggs, fish, poultry, and dairy products has little effect on your weight-control genes and spot weight loss. Even when scientists gave volunteers intravenous infusions of pure proteins in the form of amino acids, there was little gene activation.

A plethora of scientific research makes one point crystal clear: Despite the hype, protein does not play a major role in weight loss. That's why I limit protein to 20 percent of total calories.

My 7-Minute Miracle Meal plans are based on an average total intake of 1,500 calories a day. Assuming that you eat three times per day, it works out to 25 grams of protein per spot meal.

Eating platefuls of protein has become a national pastime. America has one of the highest per-capita protein consumption rates in the world. And that may not be good.

The human body has a finite limit as to how much protein it can use. Any excess protein breaks down into nitrous compounds that get processed and excreted by your kidneys.

This puts extra stress on your kidneys, forcing them to work overtime to rid the body of these protein breakdown materials.

Which country has the highest incidence of kidney disease?

The same country that eats the most protein—the United States.

Another reason not to overburden your body with mountains of protein may be premature aging. You know about anti-oxidants. These are substances like vitamins and enzymes that stabilize the internal structure of living cells. Large amounts of dietary protein can act as a pro-oxidant.

Pro-oxidants are the opposite of anti-oxidants. Pro-oxidants disrupt normal cell function and can, theoretically, hasten the aging process on the cellular level. The protein-wrinkle connection is a hot topic in medicine.

Outside of processed soy protein powder, which can reach over 90 percent purity, and egg whites (the yellow of an egg is all cholesterol) most protein-based foods are bound with fat.

Too much fat in the post-exercise meal shuts down your fat cells, something I'll talk about more when we get to fats. Though they are called "high-protein diets," don't get conned by the High-Low game. Most high-protein diets are really "high-fat diets" in disguise. You lose again.

Protein, no matter how you slice it, comes packaged with fat by nature. It may surprise you, but no matter how lean they are, no animal, fish, or poultry meat contains less than 20 percent fat.

When it comes to eating high-grade proteins, few of us are hardy or brave enough (constipation anyone?!) to eat soy or egg whites (boring!) their whole lives. Some of you can't because of allergies, others won't because of taste concerns.

The new bottom line on protein is moderation.

Twenty percent protein is fine and The 7-Minute Miracle Meal gets it right, every time.

CARBOHYDRATES: THE FAT-BURNING FAVORITE

When I hear the word carbohydrates, I think of the great Jackie Gleason crooning, "How sweeeeeet it is!"

Carbohydrates are sugars. Like them or not, carbohydrates are indispensable to life, providing immediate energy for all body functions. Your heart beats, your eyes see this page, and your brain thinks, all because of carbohydrates.

Carbohydrates are the stuff and staff of life. And death. More wars are fought over bread than protein, fat, or gold. Empires have risen and fallen on their grain reserves and will continue to do so, because hunger breeds revolution.

Right now, food drops over starving nations are mostly carbohydrates, precisely because they provide instant energy. In America, we vilify carbohydrates, but for the rest of the world, they can be precious, life-saving cargo.

It's time to welcome carbohydrates back with open arms. Why?

Because carbohydrates turn your fat cells on. That's why they are the backbone of every 7-Minute Miracle Meal. It all has to do with insulin, the carbohydrate hormone.

Insulin is directly tied into your weight-control genes. When too few carbohydrates are circulating in the blood, insulin levels fall. This lowers weight-control gene activity. The opposite—gene activation—occurs when the proper amount of carbohydrates and insulin are around.

That's why the optimal carbohydrate percentage in The 7-Minute Miracle Meal has been determined to be 50 percent. One-half of your spot meal calories come from palate-satisfying and healthy rice, potatoes, cereals, and breads.

Finally, to put a perspective on carbohydrates, consider this:

In the mid 1980's, high-carbohydrate diets were all the rage, culminating in New York Times health editor Jane Brody's bestseller: *Jane Brody's Good Food Book: Living The High-Carbohydrate* Way.

In the 1990's, they fell off the radar screen, in favor of high fat and high protein. Now, they're back again. With The 7-Minute Miracle Meal, they're here to stay.

FATS: GETTING IT JUST RIGHT

There are only two things you need to know about fat:

- Fat doesn't beget fat.
- Fat helps burn fat.

That is, the right amount of fat in the post-exercise period sure does, and that's why The 7-Minute Miracle Meal is composed of 30 percent fat.

The reasons are both scientific and practical.

Fats, like carbohydrates, are required for gene activation. But you need just the right amount. It's like Goldilocks and the Three Bears: Too little fat won't activate your weight-loss genes, but too much fat shuts them down.

On the practical side of things, fat adds one ingredient to the mix that carbohydrates and protein can't: taste.

Our perception of taste for fats is exquisite. Just the presence of a fat-containing food in your mouth is enough to stimulate hunger pangs for more. Just the sight of a sizzling fatty steak is enough to literally make your mouth water.

Fat adds flavor and texture to your food, and The 7-Minute Miracle Meal doesn't skimp on them.

FIBER: GOOD HEALTH AT BULK RATE

Any plant-based food that passes undigested through your intestines is known as fiber. There are two kinds of fiber: soluble fiber, such as vegetables, whole grains, and bran; and insoluble fiber, such as apples and citrus fruits.

They're stool bulk-builders because they hold lots of water. Apples, for instance, can absorb more than 100 times their own weight in water.

Fiber has a salutary effect on the bowels, promoting small and large intestine motility. It may help prevent gallbladder disease, colitis, and cancer of the colon.

Surprisingly, the experiments showed that fiber activates fat cells, another sound reason why you should add fiber to your diet.

EATING FOR HEALTH AND ENERGY

Each 7-Minute Miracle Meal must fulfill two goals, besides helping to burn fat from your hot spots.

First and foremost, it must promote health. Second, it should make you feel full and energetic.

You won't find anything in The 7-Minute Miracle Meal that doesn't belong in your body in the right amount. Your intake of carbohydrates, fats, and proteins must be balanced according to the formula your body has dictated.

Apparently, your body is way ahead of common lore in this area. Do you really think that nature set up your body to be a dumping ground for high-fat and high-protein diets? Think about all those globs of slimy fat trying to squeeze through your coronary arteries.

So it should be comforting to know that thousands of cardiologists agree with your food choices. Not that you'd want them all sitting at your table watching you eat. But in a sense, they are. The eating guidelines posted by the American Heart Association also suggest that we stick to the same 50/30/20 plus fiber concept. The Heart Association has come down hard on high-fat diets.

I don't know about you, but I'm glad to be on the side of thousands of doctors who hold peoples' hearts in their hands. They, of course, want to use this formula for every meal, which should be food for thought as you plan your other two meals each day.

The other main benefit of The 7-Minute Miracle Meal is that it counters one of the most chronic complaints I used to hear from patients every day: "I'm tired."

I don't hear those two words as much any more. Not once people discover the 7-minute solution. They tell me they feel energized, not fatigued.

The reason is simple: Though you may be sweaty, with cheeks rosy red, it's hard to feel tired when your heart rate is up, and blood is circulating at Daytona 500 speed. The meal that follows your exercise should augment this magical near-super-human feeling, not destroy it.

The 7-Minute Miracle Meal has enough of the right energy-rich carbohydrates to continue that post-workout glow. It has the right amount of fat to make you feel full, especially when you consider that each spot meal—including breakfast—ends with a snack.

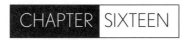

CHAPTER SIXTEEN

THE 7-MINUTE MIRACLE MEAL PLANS

It's chow time. We have twenty-one 7-Minute Miracle Meal menus for you, 7 menus each for breakfast, lunch and dinner. There's that lucky number 7 again.

Each menu gives portion sizes based on a total daily count of 1,500 calories. To make things as quick and simple as possible, brand name foods are given, so that you don't have to measure or count.

What you won't find here is a restaurant eating guide. That's because you won't find The 7-Minute Miracle Meal on the menu at your local diner. As a rule, try not to eat your spot meal out. It puts too much pressure on you.

If you know that you are going out to lunch or dinner that day, do your 7-Minute Miracle Workout in the morning and make breakfast your spot meal.

Under each menu you will find three things.

First, I've given some personal comments on the day's spot meal menu from my nearly 20 years of experience helping people lose weight. Use them to help plan your other meals for the day. You also will find an interesting collection of food and lifestyle tips, some of which may surprise you. Finally, there's a "Foods to Avoid" heading. These are foods that will gum up the works and should be avoided during the other two meals of the day. Either they contain too much fat or too many carbohydrates to fit into your 50/30/20 spot-reducing formula.

BREAKFAST

When I ask patients what they eat for breakfast, I almost always get the same answer, "Nothing. I don't eat breakfast." If I pause for a few seconds and look at them over my bifocals, they'll say "OK, I have a glass or two of orange juice, but that's it."

Again I give them the bifocal/glare routine.

"Yup, I also have two cups of coffee, with a little sugar, milk and every once in a while, a little cream."

By the time I take my glasses off, they're ready to confess.

"Sometimes, but not every morning, I'll also have a muffin and cream cheese."

It sounds like a game but it's not much fun catching a person who's in breakfast denial dead in the act. If you did a calorie count on the breakfast above, between the juice, muffin, cream cheese, milk, sugar, and occasional creamed coffee, you're almost at 800 calories!

These people have barely begun their day and already they are 800 calories in the hole.

Remember, breakfast is defined by its timing, especially if it's your spot meal for the day. My advice is to pay strict attention to the amount of food that you eat in the morning by sticking like glue to the menus. The foods to avoid also have a one- or two-word rationale. Familiarize yourself with them. But that's not to say that you can't have fun. How many of you have dessert with breakfast? Now you can. Dessert in the morning can be fun, as long as you limit it to about 100-120 calories.

In general, breakfast should be in and out. Eat and get out of the kitchen. A large, overdone breakfast is your spot-reducing nemesis. You tell your children or nieces and nephews to eat a big breakfast so that they will grow big.

You've grown enough!

LUNCH

Many people who are overweight tell me that they wouldn't dare eat what they want to while they're working. Instead, they'll have a salad and starve, sending this message to their thinner co-workers: "Look at me. I eat healthily. I don't know why I'm overweight, do you?"

When they get home, they eat like there's no tomorrow—or the day after that. The key meal for people in the workplace is lunch. Here are seven great spot lunches

Enjoy!

DINNER

In the modern American way of eating, we consume most of our calories between five and eight o'clock at night. Another way of putting it is that some of us consume 80 percent of our day's food after dark.

New research shows that parts of our brain are primed not to eat when the sun goes down, but the brain gets confused by artificial light. If this is true, then the father of modern obesity is none other than Thomas Alva Edison!

Fortunately, you don't need to be a genius to know how to eat the right way. Just follow these dinner menus.

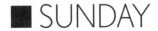

THE 7-MINUTE MEAL BREAKFAST

■ SUNDAY

1 cup Post raisin bran

¾ cup skim milk

½ cup fresh banana slices

Dessert

25 jellybeans

FOOD TO AVOID

Fried eggs. Fried bacon. Fried anything! This is one of the golden "avoid foods" for the entire program. Fried anything is out.

TODAY'S TIP

Don't stand while you're eating. Sit down and put whatever you eat on a plate. Breakfast may be a quick affair, but don't eat on the move. Studies have shown that people who eat while standing or moving eat more than they would have had they just sat down!

ABOUT TODAY'S MEAL

You must understand the yin and yang of bananas. They fill you up nicely, contain fiber, and taste great. But they will also fill you out if you eat too many. An 8 ¾-inch banana contains about 105 calories, mostly carbohydrates. Three bananas are equivalent in calories to a Snickers Bar, so don't monkey around with bananas.

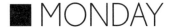

◼ MONDAY

1 cup Quaker instant oatmeal pack

1 tablespoon Kretschmer wheat germ

1 cup strawberries

¾ cup skim milk

Dessert

2 Quaker Oats Caramel Corn Cakes

FOOD TO AVOID

Kellog's Frosted Flakes. Three-quarters of a cup contains 28 grams of carbohydrates and only 1 gram of protein. That's not a great trade-off. All sugared cereals should be avoided. Though they are marketed to kids, kids and sugared cereals are not a great match.

TODAY'S TIP

Don't suck on Lifesavers. When it comes to candy, size does matter. Though they are small and contain few calories, because they are pure sugar, they encourage your pancreas to secrete insulin. Insulin in turn is a potent appetite stimulant. Use sugar-free sucking candy only.

ABOUT TODAY'S MEAL

Wheat germ is a great product that is virtually ignored by the public. Long a favorite of bodybuilders, it's got fiber *and* protein and is full of B vitamins. It also adds taste to many dishes. Try it! You'll like it!

THE 7-MINUTE MEAL BREAKFAST

■ TUESDAY

1 Thomas' oat bran English muffin

1 tablespoon Peter Pan peanut butter, smooth

1 tablespoon Polaner all fruit jam

½ cup orange juice

Dessert

1 ounce Dole trail mix

FOOD TO AVOID

Sunflower seeds. Many people start with the seed routine after breakfast assuming that because they are natural, they are good for you. Believe it or not, 1 ounce of sunflower seeds contains 160 calories and 14 grams of fat!

TODAY'S TIP

Whenever you finish taking peanut butter or jelly out of the jar, screw the cap back on and put it away and out of sight.

ABOUT TODAY'S MEAL

Orange juice must be consumed with care. When you stack up orange juice against soda, watch out! Eight ounces of Coca Cola Classic and 8 ounces of Tropicana orange juice have almost the same exact nutritional value. The vitamin C content of orange juice is negligible. Except for a half-cup in the morning, my advice is to protect yourself and your children. Stay away from the O.J.

WEDNESDAY

1 Lenders plain bagel

1 tablespoon Promise margarine spread (tub, not stick)

1 ounce Kraft natural low-fat cheddar cheese

½ pink grapefruit

Dessert

50 Keebler Mini Pretzels

FOOD TO AVOID

Lender's Big 'N Crusty Bagels. Each bagel has 240 caories and 47 grams of carbohydrates. Bagels can be tricky. Don't eat bagels from places where you don't know what's in them, like at a Dunkin' Donuts or your local diner. Some bagels have been found to contain 600 to 800 calories, without the cream cheese!

TODAY'S TIP

Brush with Rembrandt Toothpaste. This brand of toothpaste alters the acidity in the mouth and by doing so can curb your appetite after breakfast.

ABOUT TODAY'S MEAL

Low-fat cheese is cheese that has less than 5 grams of fat per ounce. Check your labels before you eat any cheese. Regular sliced cheese like Swiss, American, Muenster, and Provolone are weight-loss killers. Avoid them. Pot, cottage, and farmer's cheese are much better alternatives.

THE 7-MINUTE MEAL BREAKFAST

■ THURSDAY

1 cup Wheatena cream of wheat

1 tablespoon Promise margarine spread (tub, not stick)

1 cup skim milk

1 kiwi fruit

Dessert

2 Bachman Baked Pretzel Rods

FOOD TO AVOID

Avocado. Fruit should be analyzed case by case. Avocado is known as the "fat fruit," as one-half an avocado contains 170 calories, 130 of which come from fat!

TODAY'S TIP

Rotate the time of day that you do your 7 minutes of spot-reducing exercises. This way you'll get to try all 21 spot meals!

ABOUT TODAY'S MEAL

In this program, we only use skim milk, not whole milk. Whole milk contains too much fat. You should also be aware that low-fat dairy products may be helpful in lowering blood pressure, too.

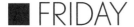 FRIDAY

2 Nutri-Grain multi-bran waffles
2 tablespoons Hungry Jack butter maple syrup, lite
1 tablespoon Promise margarine spread (tub, not stick)
1 cup skim milk
½ cup fresh blueberries
Dessert
2 graham crackers

FOOD TO AVOID

Regular calorie syrups. These can be spot-reducing killers because of
the amount of sugar they contain. Stick with our choice above. Karo
syrup, Aunt Jemima, and Log Cabin are the worst offenders. One-
quarter cup of these contains more than 200 calories and over 50
grams of carbs.

TODAY'S TIP

Many medications, including beta-blockers for high blood pressure,
antidepressants, and pain medicines, can cause weight gain. I have
seen patients gain almost 100 pounds from a medication. Be sure to
discuss weight and medication issues with a competent health professional.

ABOUT TODAY'S MEAL

Some breakfasts I can eat every day for the rest of my life. This is one
of them. Like bagels, you have to be careful with waffles. Read labels!

THE 7-MINUTE MEAL BREAKFAST

■ SATURDAY

1 scrambled egg

2 slices Arnold pumpernickel toast

1 ounce Oscar Mayer Canadian bacon

1 tablespoon Promise margarine

½ grapefruit

Dessert

2 fat-free Fig Newtons

FOOD TO AVOID

Breyers Black Cherry Yogurt. Regular yogurts are high in sugar and calories. This one has 260 calories and 50 grams of fat. I don't think of yogurt as a food. I think it's a dessert and should be avoided in the morning.

TODAY'S TIP

I saved the best for last. Chewing gum raises your metabolism enough to cause weight loss. The mechanism isn't clear, but it's worth a try, as long as you chew sugarless gum.

ABOUT TODAY'S MEAL

When eating eggs, keep in mind that the yellow is the remains of a chicken embryo and is mostly cholesterol. The white of an egg is albumin and was destined to be a growing chicken's protein source. Limit your eggs per week, or have only egg whites. And that's no yolk!

THE 7-MINUTE MEAL LUNCH

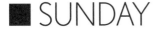 SUNDAY

2 slices Roman Meal whole-wheat bread

2 ounces Louis Rich fat-free roast turkey breast

1 tablespoon Hellmann's light mayonnaise

Lettuce leaves

Tomato slices

Dessert

$\frac{1}{2}$ cup fresh orange sections

$\frac{3}{4}$ ounce Quinlan thin pretzel sticks

FOOD TO AVOID

Cold cuts with more than 4 grams of fat per ounce. Cold cuts are also packed with salt. Be sure to check the label before you buy.

TODAY'S TIP

Many of you suffer from back pain. It's been shown that back pain can cause weight gain. To break the pain-eating cycle, see a back specialist and stay as active as you can. Oftentimes, though, back pain is a symptom of stress. Get appropriate help.

ABOUT TODAY'S MEAL

Mayonnaise is a weight-loss saboteur. Be careful. One tablespoon of Hellman's or Kraft's Real contains 100 calories and 11 grams of fat, meaning that mayonnaise is just about pure fat. Our mayonnaise choice has one-half the calories and fat.

THE 7-MINUTE MEAL LUNCH

■ MONDAY

1 cup Progresso chicken minestrone soup

2 slices Arnold pumpernickel bread

1 ounce Casbah hummus

Dessert

½ ounce Nabisco Teddy grahams vanilla snack cookies

½ cup skim milk

FOOD TO AVOID

Campbell's Tuscany Home Cookin' soup. This is mostly a salt call. Lot's wife laughs at this one! It contains twice as much salt as our choice. Too much salt is like an injection for the appetite. So be sure to check labels; many soups are basically salt with a little water.

TODAY'S TIP

Many of you rush to the health food store for the latest weight-loss supplement. The only thing that they make lighter is your bank account. Every day, patients show me labels of over-the-counter weight-loss products and ask me if I think they work. They should be asking, "Are they safe?" If you want to lose weight, stick with these meal plans. You won't find the answer in a bottle.

ABOUT TODAY'S MEAL

We used a Middle Eastern food for lunch. Don't be afraid to try foods from other countries.

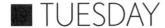

TUESDAY

Fruit and nut yogurt made with:

> 1 cup Columbo low-fat plain yogurt
>
> 1 tablespoon slivered almonds
>
> 1 tablespoon sunflower seeds
>
> 1 cup Del Monte canned peaches in juice

Dessert

> 2 Lundberg rice cakes
>
> 2 tablespoons Breakstone Temp-T-Whip cream cheese

FOOD TO AVOID

Olestra-based foods. Olestra is a synthetic fat substitute found in certain potato chips. It does nothing for you except cause weight gain, so stay away.

TODAY'S TIP

You may have heard that caffeinated green tea extract may help you shed pounds, perhaps by raising metabolism. However, the scientific proof is spotty at this point, so don't go overboard.

ABOUT TODAY'S MEAL

Almonds are part of today's fare. In general, most nuts—especially peanuts, pecans, and macadamias—are *mostly* made of fat. Be careful not to go nuts over nuts.

THE 7-MINUTE MEAL LUNCH

■ WEDNESDAY

One 2-ounce Thomas' Sahara whole wheat pita

3 ounces Bumble Bee white tuna in water

1 tablespoon Hellmann's light mayonnaise

Celery, chopped

Carrots, grated

Dessert

1 Archway No-Fat Fruit Bar cookie

1 cup skim milk

FOOD TO AVOID

Any tuna packed in oil is off-limits. It has double the calories, and a whopping ten times the fat of tuna packed in water.

TODAY'S TIP

I hate to admit this one, but diet sodas have been shown to help weight loss. I don't recommend them, but if you drink regular soda you would do well to switch to diet. Just don't overdo it.

ABOUT TODAY'S MEAL

One final comment on tuna. You may find it hard to swallow, but at certain commercial sandwich joints, a full-sized tuna sub with everything on it can pack almost 1,500 calories. Watch out, Charlie!

■ THURSDAY

3 ounces grilled chicken breast served over:

 1 cup chopped endive and radicchio

 Sliced tomato

 4 artichoke hearts in water

 $\frac{1}{2}$ cup yellow snap beans

1 tablespoon Kraft Deliciously Right Italian dressing

1 slice Arnold Cinnamon Raisin bread

1 tablespoon Promise margarine (tub, not stick)

Dessert

 1 ounce of Good & Plenty licorice candy

FOOD TO AVOID

Bernstein's Italian Dressing. It's got double the calories and double the fat of our choice

TODAY'S TIP

Sadly, some people still smoke. A study from Arizona State University shows that women who don't smoke but who are married to smokers are prone to eating fatty foods and gaining weight. So you have "second-hand weight gain" to go along with the well-documented dangers of second-hand smoke. Try and help them quit, whatever it takes.

ABOUT TODAY'S MEAL

Salad dressings are like bananas. They're fine in moderation, but overdoing them can be dangerous. Think before you pour anything on a salad. You might be better off doing it yourself, the old Italian way—vinegar and a few drops of olive oil.

THE 7-MINUTE MEAL LUNCH

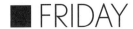 FRIDAY

Grilled vegetable wrap made with:

   18-inch Old El Paso flour tortilla

   Grilled eggplant

   Grilled onions

   Grilled zucchini

   1 ounce Kraft part skim mozzarella cheese

   1 tablespoon Mazola canola oil

Dessert

   Fruit shake made with:

   ½ cup Dole pineapple juice

   ½ cup strawberries

   ¼ banana

FOOD TO AVOID

Fried foods. I have to repeat this tip because I want you to grill your eggplant, not fry it. Again, no fried foods are permitted for any spot meal, and you should limit them at other times for health's sake.

TODAY'S TIP

Confine your food intake to your kitchen or dining room, depending on where the table is. This is a great tip to follow if you have kids, too. They learn by watching you. If you eat in front of the TV, so will they. And that can sabotage weight loss, since eating in front of the TV promotes overeating.

ABOUT TODAY'S MEAL

We went Mexican today, almost. We also used Italian partially skimmed mozzarella cheese. Whenever you eat Mexican style, avoid anything fried, as well as Monterey Jack cheese. It adds big-time fat.

■ SATURDAY

2 slices Arnold whole wheat bread

3 slices Louis Rich turkey bologna

Mustard

Tomato slices

2 Vlasic dill pickles

Dessert

1 Archway oatmeal raisin cookie

FOOD TO AVOID

Liver, brains, pancreas. There has been a return to eating organ meats. They come mostly from cows, pigs, and lambs, and are extremely fatty. Just 4 ounces of cow's pancreas, for example, contains more than 300 calories—half of which is fat!

TODAY'S TIP

I love this one. Put your fork down while you chew your food. Most people keep their fork in hand while they chew, looking down at their plate ready to harpoon their food like Captain Ahab. You'll eat less and savor it more if you take your time and put your fork down while you chew.

ABOUT TODAY'S MEAL

Today we had an Archway cookie for dessert. Cookies are tricky. Some aren't so bad, some have so much fat that they melt on the plate from your breath. I've tried them all. By far, the best all-around cookie for our purposes is Vanilla Bouquet fat-free cookies from Bakehouse Foods. They fill you up, are tasty, and are low-fat. Fabulous.

THE 7-MINUTE MEAL DINNER

■ SUNDAY

3 ounces Sockeye salmon teriyaki, broiled

⅔ cup Carolina brown rice

1 tablespoon Promise margarine spread (tub, not stick)

½ cup stir-fried snow peas

2 teaspoons Mazola canola oil (used in cooking if needed)

½ cup carrots, boiled or steamed

2 cups garden salad

2 tablespoons Kraft Deliciously Right Italian dressing

Dessert

1 cup skim milk

1 tablespoon Hershey's chocolate syrup

FOOD TO AVOID

Newman's Own Ranch Dressing. Butch and Sundance never could have gotten on their horses if they'd eaten this regularly. It's loaded with fat.

TODAY'S TIP

Dinner generates the most leftovers. And since we're all too busy to spend a lot of time in the kitchen, that's a good thing. Freeze leftovers so you have a quick, healthy meal ready when you get home late and don't feel like fixing anything.

ABOUT TODAY'S MEAL

You will often hear that salmon is fatty. It's true, but only on a relative basis. It depends on the type of fish that it's compared to. Bluefin tuna, for example, and pink salmon have nearly identical fat contents. No one is overweight because they eat too much salmon.

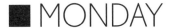 MONDAY

5 ounces shrimp, skewered and grilled with:

    Sweet red and green pepper

    Zucchini

    Mushrooms

1 tablespoon Mazola canola oil

1 cup Creamette/Penn Dutch egg noodles

1 tablespoon Promise margarine spread (tub, not stick)

Dessert

    ⅓ cup Yoplait chocolate frozen yogurt

FOOD TO AVOID

Sour cream. Think of the name, "sour cream." Don't eat any oxymorons. Use plain, low-fat yogurt instead.

TODAY'S TIP

No food should be left out on display in the kitchen. Remember what we said about visual cues and how they make your mouth water. That's why you should also zap any food-related TV commercial with the remote control, if you can find it.

ABOUT TODAY'S MEAL

Pasta isn't good for you, it's great for you. We mess up nature's best by smothering it with fatty toppings. Keep it simple. Avoid all pastas packaged as "entrees." They are super-high in fat.

THE 7-MINUTE MEAL DINNER

■ TUESDAY

Tortillas made with:

  2 Goya corn tortillas

  3 ounces ground beef, 85% lean, cooked

  6 Vlasic black olives, sliced

  1 carrot, grated

  ¼ cup Old El Paso Pico de Gallo salsa

  1 ounce Kraft natural low-fat cheddar cheese, grated

  ¾ cup Old El Paso Spanish rice, cooked

Dessert

  ½ Hostess angel food cake

FOOD TO AVOID

Rice-A-Roni Cajun Rice & Beans. I'm using this as an example of how to mess up a perfectly wonderful helping of nature's best, rice. This one has 220 calories per cup and a whopping 1,220 milligrams of salt. Avoid packaged rice entrees.

TODAY'S TIP

If you can tolerate seltzer, try drinking some with your meal. The presence of bubbles in the stomach can help curb your appetite. But as David, my 7-year-old, said, " Daddy, tell the people that they have to cover their mouths when they burp."

ABOUT TODAY'S MEAL

In today's meal, there is a great-tasting food that can garnish any salad and makes a great dip. It has 3 to 7 calories per tablespoon and zero fat. Do you give up? It's salsa!

■ WEDNESDAY

1 cup Progresso vegetable soup

3 ounces beef sirloin steak, lean, broiled

1 potato, peeled and boiled

1 tablespoon Promise margarine spread (tub, not stick)

1 cup spinach

½ cup acorn squash, cubed and boiled or steamed

Dessert

4 ounces fat-free chocolate Jell-O pudding snack

FOOD TO AVOID

Alcohol. Some people have three or four drinks in the evening: one before dinner, two during, and a nightcap. Just be aware that alcohol not only has about the same calories as fat, but also can interfere with the fat-burning process. I'm no teetotaler, but a one-drink max can't hurt.

TODAY'S TIP

I was going to save this one until the end, but I can't. Try to go to sleep on an empty stomach. Stop eating at least 3 hours before bed. And yes, that includes snacks. It's wonderful for your overall health.

ABOUT TODAY'S MEAL

Notice that you are allowed to have a chocolate-type snack. Many of us are chocoholics. When you get the urge, try our choice or a frozen chocolate pudding pop. But let's face it: Sometimes you have to have the real thing.

When you do, grab a chocolate bar. The regular size, not the giant ones. And have only one. Don't go foraging into a bag of M&M's where you won't be able to eat just one. You'll wind up eating the entire bag, just like last time.

THE 7-MINUTE MEAL DINNER

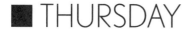

■ THURSDAY

Pasta 'n' beans made with:

  1 cup Mueller's linguini pasta, cooked

  ½ cup red kidney beans, canned

  ½ cup broccoli, chopped

  2 tablespoons Polly-O Parmesan cheese, grated

Cucumber and celery slices

2 tablespoons Kraft Deliciously Right ranch dressing

Dessert

  ½ cup Healthy Choice low-fat Cookies-and-Cream ice cream

FOOD TO AVOID

Ben & Jerry's Chocolate Cookie Dough Bar. Would you believe 420 calories? Häagen-Dazs Dark Chocolate Single. How does 400 calories grab you? By the love handles, probably.

TODAY'S TIP

For reasons unknown, most people who lose weight do so in the spring and fall. These seasons may be the time to give it your best shot.

ABOUT TODAY'S MEAL

Ice cream is an emotional food. It conjures up childhood memories because more often than not it was used as a reward food. Many patients tell me that they keep containers of it in the freezer for their own children. There is a lesson here that adults should learn.

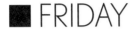 FRIDAY

Tofu stir-fry made with:

- 1/2 cup Silken extra-firm tofu
- 1/4 cup sautéed scallops
- 1 cup Chinese cabbage, stir-fried
- 2 ounces water chestnuts
- 1/2 cup Green Giant vegetable almond stir-fry
- 1 cup Nasoya rice noodles

Dessert

- 1 Archway carrot cake cookie

FOOD TO AVOID

Fruit juice. Though we covered orange juice in the Breakfast section, fruit juice in general stacks up poorly to soda, especially in terms of calories and sugar. When you have a moment, sit down with a can of Coke Classic and your favorite fruit juice and see for yourself.

TODAY'S TIP

Stay away from salad bars and buffets. Signs that promise "All-you-can-eat" are like detour signs on the road to weight loss. When you see one, here's what it should tell you: Road closed.

ABOUT TODAY'S MEAL

Today we had some stir-fried Chinese cabbage. When it comes to cooking techniques, the best are stir-frying, steaming, grilling, poaching, roasting, or boiling. And I'll say it one more time: almost anything but fried. But by now, you know that, don't you?

THE 7-MINUTE MEAL DINNER

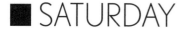 ## SATURDAY

3 ounces chicken breast, covered with 2 tablespoons Post bran flakes, ground
with any spice for flavor and then baked

½ cup mashed sweet potato

6 asparagus spears

½ cup Birds Eye International vegetables

1 tablespoon Promise margarine spread (tub, not stick)

Dessert

½ cup Healthy Choice low-fat chocolate chip ice cream

FOOD TO AVOID

Swanson Hungry Man Chicken Dinner. This one has 690 calories and almost 1,400 milligrams of salt. It's not much different from other TV chicken dinners. Stay away.

TODAY'S TIP

Stay out of the kitchen unless you have official business there, like fixing a meal or eating. It shouldn't be used as a den or playroom. Don't watch TV there, and kids shouldn't be doing their homework there.

ABOUT TODAY'S MEAL

We used bran flakes to make chicken. That reminds me that one fun weight-loss trick is to reverse breakfast and dinner every once in a while. Have cereal for dinner, and meat or fish for breakfast. Sometimes that tricks the appetite center in the brain and you feel full on less food.

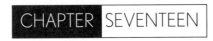

CHAPTER SEVENTEEN

MAKING YOUR OWN 7-MINUTE MIRACLE MEAL

I've given you specific menus for every day of the week. But at some point, you're going to want to try something a little different. That's okay. I'm not about to tell you to eat the same seven spot meals for the rest of your life.

Fortunately, putting together your own 7-Minute Miracle Meal is a cinch.

After all, we're only talking about one meal per day! And you don't need a bachelor's degree in nutrition. You can use you master's degree in common sense, instead.

The average American supermarket is stocked with 14,000 items, three times more than in 1960. Though it sometimes seems like you've tried all 14,000 at one sitting, in reality it's impossible for you to be familiar with them all.

You don't have to be. You already know the formula for the ideal 7 Minute Miracle Meal:

- 50 percent carbohydrates
- 30 percent fat
- 20 percent protein
- Fiber

These percentages are based on a total calorie count of between 500 and 600 calories per post-exercise meal. You know from my menu plans which foods work and which don't. So determining the correct composition for your own meals should be just a matter of reading labels.

It should be. But these days, foods are plastered with labels like travel stickers on old steamer trunks. I understand that it all can get so confusing that you feel lost.

Here's a different approach.

GET YOURSELF ON THE "A" LIST

I'm going to give you two 7-Minute Miracle Meal master lists to work from.

First comes the "A" list.

The "A" list contains the perfect post-exercise food choices, either because they are comprised of 30 percent total fat calories or less, or because they contain the right amount of carbohydrates and protein to energize your weight-control genes.

Not only are these foods low in fat, some contain no fat at all!

If most of your choices come from the "A" list, you won't go astray.

As for desserts, you already have close to thirty of them in The 7-Minute Miracle Meal menus in the preceding chapters that you can rotate among breakfast, lunch, and dinner. But if you need more, I'll share with you my one personal, all-time favorite. It's a killer.

STAY OFF THE "F" LIST

The second list is the "F" list. "F" as in fat = failure.

If you want to succeed, stay away from any foods that made the "F" list because too many of their total calories come from fat. The easiest way to screw up your 7-Minute Miracle Meal is to eat too much fat.

Big-time fat negates your 7-Minute Miracle Workout, big-time. You may be surprised to find that some of your favorite foods are on the "F" list. Keep in mind that The 7-Minute Miracle Meal is just that: one meal. It's what you eat 40 minutes after your workout. The rest of the day you may eat as you normally do, including foods from the "F" list, provided you do so in moderation.

Do you remember the funky robot from the great TV show and horrible movie, *Lost In Space?* When it sensed a threat, it gyrated, beeped, flashed its lights, and blared: "Danger, Will Robinson, Danger! Danger!"

That's the warning that your own spot-reducing robot would shout if you eat mass quantities of foods from the "F" list. And, of course, if your name happened to be Will Robinson.

Speaking of mass quantities, use the same portions in the meal you devise for yourself as provided in my menu plan. If you choose a different breakfast cereal, fish entrée, or dessert than the one I recommend, be sure to stay close to the portion sizes of comparable foods listed.

Foods from both the "A" and "F" lists are presented from best to worst, depending on what percentage of fat calories they contain.

The "A" list begins with foods that have 0 percent fat. As you climb the fat ladder, you eventually arrive at those "F" list foods that are 100 percent fat, such as butter and lard.

THE "A" LIST

■ FOODS WITH LITTLE OR NO FAT

The energy-rich foods below contain very little fat. Some have no fat. Most are carbohydrates except for egg whites, which are mostly protein. (The yellow part of an egg is mostly cholesterol.)

Eat your carbohydrates au natural, as close to how nature provides them as possible. Don't drown them in butter, oil, sauces, or dressings.

For example, vegetables taste great raw, or with some balsamic vinegar or non-fat dressing. Covering them with fatty, oily dressings and bacon bits destroys their wholesomeness and your spot-reducing potential.

The ideal post-workout meal calls for 50 percent carbohydrates, so when you look down at your plate, roughly one-half of it should be filled with choices from this list:

- Pasta
- Beans
- Potatoes
- Vegetables
- Dry cereal
- Bread
- Dry cottage cheese
- Rice
- Fruit
- Egg whites
- Skim milk

■ FOODS LESS THAN 20 PERCENT FAT

Most of your protein sources should come from this list:

- Crab
- Shrimp
- Lobster
- Tuna in water
- Low-fat cottage cheese
- Most broiled fish
- Sliced skinless white turkey
- Roasted skinless chicken

■ FOODS THAT ARE 20 PERCENT TO 30 PERCENT FAT

These five foods sneak in just under the "A" list cutoff:

> ## My Favorite Dessert
>
> Here is one incredible "A" list dessert. It not only tastes great and is low in fat, but it will fill you up like there's no tomorrow. It's Silhouette's Fat-Free Fudge Bars. Silhouette, which specializes in low-fat and fat-free ice cream products, is located in New York and has its own web site, www.skinnycow.com.
>
> And in case you're skeptical, no, I have no connection with the company whatsoever. I just love this mouthwatering treat. When you see one, hold it, and taste it, you'll ask yourself the same question that I do each time I have one: "How can something this big and sweet have only 60 calories, without a single one coming from fat?"

- Low-fat yogurt
- Veal rib
- 2 percent low-fat milk
- Rump cuts

■ FIBER

By design, most of the carbohydrates that make up The 7-Minute Miracle Meal are already rich in fiber. So you don't have to go out of your way to find more. Here are some smart and tasty choices to boost your fiber intake:

- Beans
- Peas
- Dried fruits, such as raisins and apricots
- Cereals
- Brown rice
- Potatoes
- Lentils
- Nuts

THE "F" LIST

The foods on this list are on notice. They are the ones that you have to watch out for when preparing your own 7-Minute Miracle Meal.

■ FOODS 35 PERCENT TO 50 PERCENT FAT

At first glance, some of these foods don't seem that bad because their fat contents are not that outrageous. But these foods also are loaded with calories, which is bad news when you try to stick to the 500-600 calorie limit of The 7-Minute Miracle Meal.

In addition, this group is a sugar goldmine. Dumping high-sugar foods on your body causes the hormone insulin to rise in your blood. High levels of insulin, in turn, can shut down the fat-burning process.

- Ice cream
- Crackers
- Cold cuts
- Cookies
- Cake
- Donuts
- Flank beef

■ FOODS 50 PERCENT TO 65 PERCENT FAT

These foods should be excluded from any post-exercise meal:

- Pork loin
- Ground beef
- Canned ham
- Veal cutlet
- Rib steak
- Skim milk cheeses
- Chicken with skin

■ FOODS 65 PERCENT TO 80 PERCENT FAT

Most of the foods in this section are not only high in fat, they also are loaded with salt. Too much salt has a tendency to make you hungry. Leave these foods alone after you exercise:

- Swiss cheese
- Blue cheese
- Muenster cheese
- American cheese
- Cheddar cheese
- Hot dogs
- Tuna in oil
- Prime rib
- Pork chop
- Potato chips
- Liverwurst
- Herring

■ FOODS 80 PERCENT TO 90 PERCENT FAT

I'll bet that you'll find some surprises in this list. You won't believe how high in fat some of these are.

After all, aren't foods such as sesame seeds and peanuts touted as "healthy" at health-food stores? Yes, they are, and with some justification. (Sunflower seeds aren't that great, either!) But that's not the issue. Again, it's not that you should avoid these completely. Just don't eat them as part of your daily 7-Minute Miracle Meal.

And think twice before you smother your bagel with cream cheese, pour an avalanche of salad dressing on your salad, down a handful of pistachios, or open that can of tuna in oil. Don't let the commercial trappings of these foods trap you: They are a fat trap.

- Regular calorie salad dressing
- Cream cheese
- Sesame seeds
- Corned beef
- Avocados
- Almonds
- Pistachios
- Sausage
- Walnuts

■ FOODS MORE THAN 90 PERCENT FAT

These foods are almost pure fat. And nothing will sabotage your 7-Minute Miracle Meal faster. So don't even think about adding these to your supermarket cart. Just walk on by.

- Butter
- Baking chocolate
- Lard
- Cream
- Cooking and salad oils
- Mayonnaise
- Bacon
- Vegetable shortening

PART THREE

WHAT ARE YOU DOING THE REST OF YOUR LIFE?

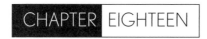

CHAPTER EIGHTEEN

KEEPING IT OFF FOR GOOD!

They say that the shortest measurable span of time is the nanosecond between when a light changes from red to green in a Times Square intersection and when the cab driver behind you leans on his horn.

And the second-shortest time span?

It's the 3 milliseconds that elapse between finishing a consultation with a new patient before that patient asks: "But Dr. Levine, what happens when I stop the program? Will my thighs come back?"

They haven't even started and they're already worried about stopping. What about you? Are you concerned about your own prospects for long-term weight loss? Did you ever lose weight, only to have every single pound—and then some—return later?

Most of us have. And that's how we learned a valuable, but daunting, lesson: Losing weight and keeping weight off are two different things.

Keeping weight off is much harder.

MIND OVER MAINTENANCE

There is no longer any doubt that potent genetic forces are at play here. For years, scientists have been searching for a maintenance factor—the "M" factor, if you will—a way to give people who have lost weight at least a fighting chance to keep it off.

They found not one, but two. Can you guess what two things you need to do to succeed over the long haul? No, it's not willpower. And no, you don't have to be a champion dieter. Stuffing your face with protein until it comes out of your ears doesn't cut it, either.

How about dividing your food intake into five or six smaller meals instead of three squares? Uh-uh.

None of these matter because the first "M" factor is not something that you eat or don't eat

It's how you think.

A recent study involving a group of psychiatrists who interviewed scores of people who were successful at long-term weight loss produced fascinating results.

This was a double-blind study, the gold standard of scientific investigation. The psychiatrists and the study subjects not only had never met each other before, but neither group even knew what the study was about.

Later, the aim of the study was revealed: To determine if there is one mental or personality trait that gives the successful long-term, weight-loss candidate an advantage over others.

The shrinks were then asked to use one word to describe the people they interviewed, to see if that word would tell them something about the elusive success factor.

And the word that they came up with most often?

Fanatical.

You see, long-term weight changes in your body begin upstairs between your ears. You have to be at the top of your game mentally and feeling really good about yourself before the physical changes take place.

Does this mean you need to ratchet your enthusiasm up to fanatical level?

No, but a steadfast commitment to your plan of action is a must.

If you are grasping for one diet, then another, like Tarzan reaching for the next swinging vine, there is a good chance that you haven't found yourself, commitment-wise, yet.

Commitment means staying a course and making a plan work.

Of course, if the demands of a particular weight-loss plan are unreasonable—such as eating only fats or proteins, or sticking to an 800-calorie-a-day diet—then the plan itself doesn't warrant commitment.

That's why you have a distinct advantage.

The 7-Minute Miracle asks you to work out for a few minutes a day, followed by a meal based on the guidelines of the American Heart Association.

That's not only reasonable, it's doable, eminently doable.

So do it.

Speaking of doing it, when you do your 7-minute workout on a regular basis, you bring the other "M" factor into play. Because regular exercise *is* the other "M" factor.

Working out consistently thwarts regaining pounds after weight loss. That's a fact, proved multiple times in multiple studies. Amazingly, we don't understand how exercise does what it does and we don't know how much or how little you have to do!

We do know that it's got nothing to do with burning calories, because the studies showed that far fewer calories were expended than are required to keep weight off. And I do know this: Show me someone who can't maintain their weight loss, and I'll show you someone who doesn't exercise on a regular basis.

FAT CELLS NEVER FORGET

I once asked a patient if he jogged.

"Me, jog?" he replied, incredulously. "The only thing that I jog in the morning is my memory."

Another jokingly said, "Yeah, I exercise every morning. I exercise my right to stay in bed."

I hear variations on these two a lot, along with, "I wrestle every day—with my conscience over whether I should exercise or not."

When it comes to exercise, everyone's a comedian. It's a natural defense mechanism to deflect attention away from the simple fact that they're not doing something they know they should be doing.

Sometimes, patients tell me that they can't remember the last time they exercised. That's okay. They don't need to have clear memories, because their fat cells, like elephants, never forget.

Your computer has memory and so do your fat cells. They remember what it was like in the good old days when they were filled to the brim with fat. You can almost picture those microscopic blobs of fat singing, "Misty watercolor memories, of the way we were..."

No matter how much fat you lose from your belly or tush, a certain fraction of your fat cells are serenading your hot spots with a heartfelt version of "The Way We Were." That's because your weight-control genes are like a broken record. They just want to keep the fat cells of your belly, butt, thighs, hips, and arms full of fat.

It's time to put a new record on your body's jukebox: "Hit the Road, Fat."

Putting your body in motion and keeping it *going and going and going* like the Energizer bunny for 7 minutes is enough to change your fat cells' tune.

On the microscopic level this may be due to an increase in lipase activity inside your fat cells. Lipase is the enzyme inside fat cells that helps break down fat. Usually, it's about as active as Al Gore on the dance floor. Exercise, over the long haul, energizes your fat cells. Think James Brown, in his prime.

Should you stop exercising for any length of time, lipase goes back to sleep once more, prodding your cells to open up to take in new fat deposits.

What does all this tell you about exercise?

Don't stop!

DAY 1, DAY 1,000

Most weight-loss programs have elaborate, complicated maintenance schedules with enough rules and regulations to make the most anal-retentive government bureaucrat proud.

Not us. It can't get any easier than this.

Whatever you do on day 1—a 7-minute workout, followed by a 40-minute pause and a delicious meal—is exactly the same thing you'll do on day 100, day 1,000, or day 10,000. Make The 7-Minute Miracle's Genetic Body Sculpting Plan part of your daily routine and you're in business.

It's that simple.

Spending 7 minutes exercising and waiting 40 minutes to eat afterwards is hardly a steep price to pay for holding on to the new slimmer you. And the daily 7-Minute Miracle Meal? You have to eat anyway, so you might as well eat to lose!

With a plan this simple, why would you ever want to stop? Just keep on going, and going, and going, and going ...

NO MORE EXERCUSES!

As a board-certified realist, I know that although the evidence that regular exercise plays a big role in weight-loss maintenance is undeniable, your desire to find an easy way out may be stronger.

Perhaps you still think of exercise as a chore. Like other chores, exercise winds up on a list of things that should be done, but never are, under the heading "Excuses Not To Exercise." For most of us, it's a long list.

I call these excuses not to exercise *exercuses*. They all begin with three words, *I am too* ...tired ... busy ... hot ... cold ... sleepy ... sickly ... stuffy ... depressed ... stressed ... achy ... (fill in your own favorite here).

I've heard 'em all before.

Once or twice a week, patients even hand me the ultimate exercise: "I hate exercise."

Sharron H. a 38-year-old recently separated computer consultant, told me: "Exercise? I hated it in high school. I hated it in college. I hated it when I was single. I hated it when I was married. And now that I'm single again, I hate it again."

Sharron's hardly alone. Fewer than 5 percent of overweight Americans exercise vigorously on a regular basis, and fewer than 15 percent do any exercise at all. Those of you who feel this way but still want spot-reducing results for life, need a change of heart.

A CHANGE OF HEART

I admit that when the North Jersey winter waits outside to freeze my bones to icicles, but it's sizzling-griddle-cakes-warm under my blankets, forget exercise, I don't want to move.

I admit that sometimes in steamy August, mega-drops of congealed humidity choke off my trachea, making me want to stay home and suck the air out of my air conditioner.

On days like these, exercise is as appealing as dinner with your ex-boss, but I make it to the gym anyway. Ken M., my trainer, is going to be there, that I know for sure.

Maybe you and I need a change of heart, but Ken doesn't. He already had a change of heart—someone else's.

When Ken was only 2 months old, he had his first of seven open-heart operations for severe congenital heart disease. How many 6-year-olds do you know with a ventricular pacemaker generator implanted in their abdomens?

How many 6-year-olds do you know who must wear a bulletproof vest while playing to protect his chest in case he falls?

As the years passed, Ken's damaged heart muscles continued to weaken. In June of 1997, Ken married Susan, but while he was on his honeymoon, he became so tired, sweaty, and so gasping for air that he couldn't leave his hotel room.

For most of us, that may sound two ceiling mirrors short of an ideal honeymoon. But for Ken, it meant that his heart and his lungs were failing. Badly.

A few weeks later, Ken received a heart transplant at Columbia Presbyterian Medical Center in New York City. From that point on, Ken had to add eight rejection medicines to the seven meds he already took for his cardiovascular system.

Unfortunately, the gods of ill health weren't quite through with him, and one of Ken's rejection drugs thinned and ruined the top part of his hip bones, causing the same hip problem—bone necrosis—that forced the great professional athlete Bo Jackson to retire prematurely.

In 1998, Ken underwent a painful bone graft to correct his hip condition. Today, he looks and feels terrific, and works fulltime as an enthusiastic certified personal trainer. Ken works out hard, headphones on, in his own world, pushing his body.

By the way, he never tells his clients his own story and just about no one in the gym (until now!) knows what you now know.

I hope you caught the lesson here. This is not a network sob story with a happy ending. It's not a story to inspire you, either, because while Ken is my personal trainer, I don't seek his inspiration. What I want from him is perspiration!

You won't find him sitting lazily on some exer-cycle machine reading the *Bergen Record* newspaper, or going through the motions with a featherweight dumbbell. At every session, he works out with a wave of intensity that I try to catch for my own workouts, no matter how "not into it" I feel that day. Intensity is contagious!

But that's not the essence of this story either.

The real story here is about genes.

Though his body was put through nature's genetic wringer, Ken doesn't allow his genetics to tell him what he can and can't do. He doesn't use the bad genetic hand he was dealt at birth as an excuse. He uses it as a starting point.

If your thighs, hips, or butt are too beefy, do something about them. If the back of your arms jiggle like jelly, get moving. If you have too much flab on your abs, get busy.

Work at it.

Sweat.

Sweat some more.

Then work even harder.

And the next time you find yourself running down your long list of exercises, trying to find just the right one to match the way you feel that day, remind yourself that it's the 6 inches between your breast bone and your backbone that counts most.

When you exercise, don't just show up.

Put your heart into it!

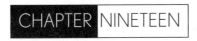

CHAPTER NINETEEN

WE DID IT ...
SO CAN YOU!

If there are 5 billion people on this planet, this guy I've known my whole life is stronger than four billion nine hundred ninety nine million nine hundred thousand (and change) of them, give or take one or two weightlifters from Mongolia.

Yet he never understood that to look good, he had to have less body fat, not bigger muscles. He was in definition denial.

By his own estimation, over his adult life, he worked out for a total of 65,000 hours, lifting tons of weight each *hour*! By closely following the workouts of old bodybuilding pros like Dave Draper, Bill Pearl, and Larry Scott, he was able—at 6-foot, 2-inches—to bulk up and compete in bodybuilding contests along the East Coast (including Mr. Apollo, Mr. Manhattan, Mr. Brooklyn, and Mr. Delaware, Mr. Maryland, and Mr. Virginia). He even earned special trophies for his abdominal musculature.

Fast-forward 25 years.

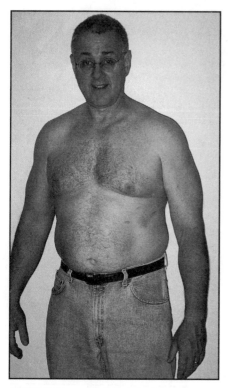

BEFORE: Time turns a bodybuilder into body blubber!

The photo below shows how time can turn a bodybuilder into a body blubber.

But looks can be deceiving. Under that thick coating of blubber are powerful muscles, strong enough to win or place in scores of power-lifting competitions, including the World II Bench Press Championships and the Atlantic Coast Championships, as well as the New Jersey and New York State Bench Press Championships.

Today, at age 51 and weighing 200 pounds, this guy is capable of

1. Bench pressing 400 pounds.
2. Squatting 500 pounds.
3. Doing 10 full pushups with a 220-pound man standing on his back.
4. Dipping 5 times with a 150-pound dumbbell attached to him.
5. Curling 200 pounds with two hands.
6. Wrist-curling 100 pounds with one hand.

These are considered world-class, drug-free, age-correlated lifts. Yet, his big belly sabotaged what potentially could have been a pleasing physique. The best abdominals in town declined over time to the worst gut on the block.

Frankly, I'm surprised he had the courage to furnish the photos for this book. Forgive me if you think I'm making fun of this poor guy.

I'm not. I'm just being realistic.

The guy in the pictures is me.

PUTTING MYSELF ON THE SPOT

Despite grueling 2- to 3-hour workouts, my "six-pack" abs turned into "two six-packs a day" abs. But walking around with a big belly wasn't the worst of it. The really bad news was what was happening inside my belly.

My hot spot was really hot, because my type of abdominal fat is heart attack fat.

I couldn't imagine anything worse. My own body fat, like a cancer, could kill me. But it's true. Somehow, I thought that nature should reward, not punish, me for all the time I put in sweating it out in dungeons disguised as gyms around the world.

But a closer look at my own family tree revealed that I was becoming a victim of my own genetics. I had the same big belly as my father, who later developed diabetes and had a heart attack.

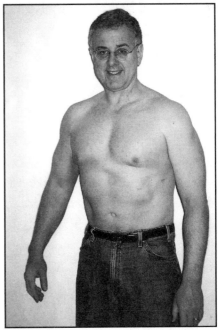

I had to face the truth. I was not immune to the powerful role that genetics plays in weight gain. No one is. Forget how bad I looked. My 43-inch belly was unhealthy.

I needed my old abs back!

But how? It wasn't a question of exercise, because I was already exercising to the max. If I dieted, I probably could lose a few inches of belly fat, but I would also lose muscle tissue and strength, and that's not an option for me.

So I changed course.

Spurred on by the new re-

AFTER: From six-pack-a-day abs to a nice six-pack!

search in gene science, I concentrated on getting rid of my belly fat, not building bigger abdominal muscles.

Though it went against everything I was taught in school and in my years as a strength athlete, I spot-reduced my belly without compromising other body parts. And I'm healthier for it.

When I started, I never imagined that I could eat and exercise my belly away. But as you can see from the new photo below, my abs have shrunk from 43 inches to 34 inches. This is a natural picture. I am not flexing, holding my breath, or trying to gather my stomach in.

To paraphrase the TV ads, I not only developed The 7-Minute Miracle. I'm also the first customer.

Tired of having a big belly, I finally got it right, and so will you.

What worked for me to trim 9 inches off my midsection is the same 7-minute abdominal workout on page 108, followed by the 40-minute pause and post-exercise 7-Minute Miracle Meal.

If you notice, I also lost my love handles. The waist and abdominal muscles share many blood vessels, so it's not surprising that both can be trimmed at the same time.

I also should mention that my father is doing well, and today he has the same 32-inch waist he had playing college football 60 years ago. The first thing he does when he gets out of bed is to do one pushup for every year of his age.

This morning he did 82!

No matter which of the five hot spots is your bane, you are miles ahead of where I started on the learning curve because you already know that spot weight loss is based on breaking down fat, not gaining muscle.

GETTING THE LEAD OUT

I developed this program for those of you who don't enjoy lifting weights.

Of course, if you do lift weights, don't stop. I didn't. Just know that weightlifting will not shrink your hot spots. Though I am proud of the weightlifting trophies that crowd my office, I realize that "hoisting lead" is not the exercise option for everyone.

The 7-Minute Miracle works without you having to venture within a mile of a gym. Maybe even 10 miles.

REAL PEOPLE, REAL STORIES

I've told you all about the science behind The 7-Minute Miracle. But I'm living proof that this program doesn't just work in a lab. It works in real life. For real people, just like you.

Here are the true stories of four other people who have used The 7-Minute Miracle to reshape their body contours. I chose these four individuals out of the many who follow The 7-Minute Miracle program because they are easy to relate to and they illustrate points particular to genetic body sculpting.

All four share a common genetic thread. Though none are related, genes play a definite role in their stories.

For men, the focus is on their number one hot spot: the belly.

It amazes me how many women describe their significant others as having a slight paunch. Yet, when I meet the men in their lives, inevitably you can barely fit a piece of paper between their hanging bellies and the floor! Okay, I exaggerate—a little. I guess it only goes to show that love truly is blind.

None of these case histories involve massive weight losses. None are about women who were once obese but are now fashion models.

The average American woman stands 5-foot 4, and weighs about 146 pounds. The average professional model stands 5-foot 9, and weighs 119 pounds. (Twiggy, the 1960's British supermodel, stood 5-foot 7, and weighed 92 pounds.) The chasm between real women and professional models is wider than the Grand Canyon, and will always be.

That doesn't bother us, though, because spot reducing is not about chasing a number on a scale.

Spot weight loss is about changing *your* contours and improving *your* muscular definition. It's about shrinking *your* hot spots. Don't worry about what some fashion model is doing. She has her genes and her jeans, you have yours!

The images in the before and after photos speak for themselves. When you examine the photos, I want you to look not only *at* the photos, I want you to look *through* the photos to a deeper level. Think about what's going on inside, not just outside. Think of how these people came to terms with their own fat cells and weight-control genes.

That has made all the difference.

See for yourself.

A 7-MINUTE SUCCESS

■ LISA S., 31

BIG BACKSIDES ARE A FAMILY AFFAIR

A woman walking down the street finds a magic lamp, which she promptly rubs. Out comes a genie who offers to grant her any wish. "I wish that my tush were smaller," she answers.

The genie, dismayed by her request, asks: "What about all of the other people around the world with problems?"

"Fine," the woman answered, spreading her arms out wide. "I wish that *everyone* in the world had a smaller tush."

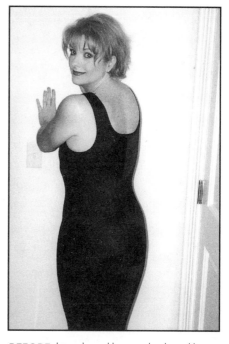

BEFORE: Lisa shared her mother's and her sister's genes, so her tush couldn't fit in her favorite jeans.

I love that one. And that's exactly what Lisa S., a mother of two from Bergen County, New Jersey, wanted: a smaller butt.

Lisa stands 5-foot 5 and weighs 152 pounds. This puts her in the slightly overweight category by current weight-loss standards, but Lisa's true weight problem began and ended at the seat of her pants.

I'll let her speak for herself:

■

My backside began to sprout the split second that I conceived my second daughter, Amy. Not that it was so great before, but at least I was only in a slightly self-conscious mode.

Once Amy arrived, it was adios, self-conscious, and hello, self-absorbed. Like when I'm on line at the supermarket, I'm worrying that not only is every one in the building staring at my backside, they're using night vision goggles to get a better look!

ALL IN THE FAMILY

My tush is a family affair.

When I look in the mirror, I see three people: my mother, my sister, and me. Not only are all of our backsides the same size, they're the same shape. When any of us would drop a couple of pounds, which wasn't often, our backsides wouldn't change for beans.

And believe me, I've tried everything.

My friend Laurie e-mailed me this great diet that was big in Southern California, promising 10 pounds off in 10 days. I've fallen for this stuff before, but I know myself. I need quick results to stay motivated.

The great West Coast plan turned out to be the same 600-calorie, soup-and-juice diet that I lost 6 pounds with the week before cheerleader try-outs. I hated it 15 years ago. I couldn't stomach doing it now.

I did the high protein thing at least a zillion times. The last ended the instant that I smelled the Pizza at Enzo's, a local Italian trattoria, 48 hours later.

I combined foods. I juiced. I ate six small meals, each bigger than the one before. I joined the center where you watch your weight ... again. I've been there so many times that I was invited to the leader's daughter's sweet sixteen! Two behemoth Dunkin' Donut Bavarian Creams ended my latest attempt.

Of course, I didn't just try dieting. I've been through the Full exercise Monty, too.

One night, reinforced by a few glasses of Merlot, I got on a friend's treadmill. In the weird shadows of the dull yellow basement light, it looked like "the rack"—not my favorite medieval torture machine.

I lasted only 2 minutes. I never last more than 2 minutes. Running and sweating on top of a revolving black rubber carpet reminds me way too much of a guinea pig running on a plastic wheel in a cage. Come by our next garage sale and the treadmill is yours for a fiver.

Then I joined a big-name gym. It had all the bells and whistles, like the Dead Sea mud treatments, a tanning salon, spinning, massage therapy, and stretching classes. Up front was a nutrition bar, stocked with supplements, protein drinks, energy bars, fat blockers, fat emulsifiers, fat grabbers, and bottles with labels that had 20 to 30 ingredients.

Regardless of the ingredients, they all had two things in common: They did nothing for me and they tasted terrible.

And of course they had weights, tons of them. I already had a full-time job and lifting and pumping anything sounded too much like another job to me. So I joined a kick-boxing cardio class, "Great Glutes," that met three times a week. After 3 months, I lost 2 pounds, but my rump still trailed behind like a concrete shadow.

Elayne, my best friend, told me about Joe, a personal trainer. So I hired him. Six weeks passed, and I lost nothing. In our next-to-last encounter, I complained that nothing had changed and my butt was stuck exactly where it was before we started.

"Lisa, don't worry," Joe said. "Your backside is all muscle and a pound of muscle weighs more than a pound of fat"

How lame is that one? I'm no nuclear physicist, but even I know that 1 pound of any substance weighs exactly the same as 1 pound of any other substance, at least here on the planet earth!

While my buns stayed, Joe had to go.

Oh, one more thing.

You know that Walkman-sized electronic muscle stimulator advertised on TV that trims your abs? Well, I thought I was a genius by turning it around to stimulate my butt! Fortunately, it was too small to be noticed. Unfortunately, it didn't stimulate anything ... except for my imagination.

■

Lisa is a riot and a real straight-shooter. Her story reminds me of Yogi Berra's response when the Yankees lost the 1960 World Series to the Pittsburgh Pirates: "We made too many wrong mistakes!"

Many of you probably nodded your head in recognition as you read Lisa's story. She recognized early on that her problem spot was genetic and became more of a problem after she gave birth. Yet, she was willing to keep trying different diets and exercises because she blamed herself for making too many wrong mistakes.

I told her that she didn't make *any* mistakes.

Everything she tried was from the BG Era—*Before Gene*. We are now in the AG Era—*After Gene*.

Genes don't like starvation or high-protein (a.k.a. high-fat) diets. As for the exercises Lisa

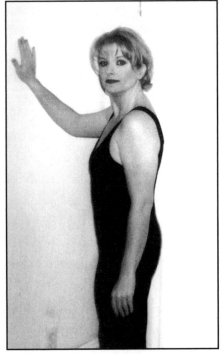

AFTER: Lisa in the After-Gene (AG) Era. Now she's ready for a new, smaller, pair of jeans.

tried, they either targeted muscle tissue and not fat, or they didn't stimulate her weight-control genes.

It didn't take but a drop of extra cajoling to get Lisa to try the 7-minute butt workout on page 86, followed by the 40-minute, no-eating pause and a spot meal.

She's now big into the idea of burning fat for 6 or 7 hours after she exercises. Paul Simon says there are 50 ways to leave your lover, but he doesn't say which one works best. The same is true for most weight-loss programs.

This is what Lisa looks like now.

After years of trying, Lisa found what works best for her. And it only takes her 7 minutes a day.

A 7-MINUTE SUCCESS

■ DEBBIE R., 30

LEARNING TO LOVE EXERCISE IN 7 MINUTES

Until her tenth high school reunion, Debbie R. still thought of herself as the slim young girl who members of the basketball team used to love to dance with at school dances.

Sure, she had gained 6 pounds, but she didn't give them much thought. Until a tactless comment by an old boyfriend at the reunion caused her to change the way she looked at herself.

After a few drinks, her old flame reminisced about how her waist used to be so small in high school that—with one outstretched hand—the players could almost hold her lower back from one side to the other, palming it, like a basketball.

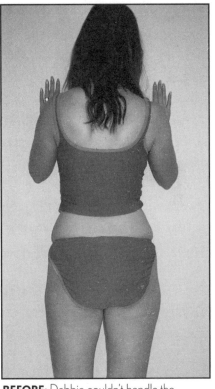

BEFORE: Debbie couldn't handle the "premature middle-age spread" that gave her "love handles."

He then went on to assure Debbie that she shouldn't worry that she had put on a few pounds. After all, he said, so had many of her classmates. He then opened his blazer to reveal a burgeoning beer belly. How attractive!

Debbie, who travels a great deal selling radio advertising, came to the sudden realization that she had developed "premature middle-age spread," a phrase she coined herself.

It's amazing. One comment made her age a decade.

But these were no ordinary 6 pounds. They were, she imagined, 6 pounds of marshmallows bunched around her waist.

Here is what Debbie looked like when I first saw her.

You can see her problem area for yourself. Not horrendous by any standard, but she definitely had developed love handles. Debbie asked me to give her a diet so she could lose her hips in "two or three weeks" before her next business trip to Texas.

I asked Debbie if anyone in her family had hip issues. "Yes, my mother and two aunts have problems *just like mine*," she replied.

I explained to her that her hips aren't *like* her mother's and aunts,' they *are* her mother's and aunts.' A large hip size was a shared genetic family trait and Debbie is the latest heir.

After a spirited discussion in which we both agreed that fad diets cannot prevail against her genes. I explained that, in reality, not even the 7-Minute Miracle meal would get rid of her hot spot, unless it's preceded by 7 minutes of fat-targeting exercises.

Debbie, ever the anti-exercise diehard, balked at the thought of even a 7-minute workout. Like an arthritic mule, she wouldn't budge.

That's when I let it all hang out.

I took off my stethoscope, hit the carpet and started doing the three hip-busting exercises found on page 91.

She got the less than subtle hint and tried them, too. To her credit she lasted about 2½ minutes, finishing all sweaty, out of breath, and giggling! I even hooked her up to an electrocardiograph machine so she could have a graphic record of her elevated heart rate.

I wish I had a tape recorder to capture her laughter because Debbie couldn't believe that she was actually having a good time exercising. That's because for the first time in years, she got to feel her own adrenaline pumping.

Afterwards, we talked about the importance of exercise intensity over exercise duration. Suddenly, 7 minutes wasn't such a big, bad, barrier.

Debbie's impromptu decision to try The 7-Minute Miracle Workout turned her into a believer. Selling her on the 40-minute pause and the spot meal were cake compared to motivating this anti-exerciser.

You cannot spot reduce without paying your 7-minute dues. For those of you who aren't into moving your body, many experts advise that you start out walking and perhaps gradually build up from there.

No way!

You will never learn how to swim, if you walk laps around the pool. Jump in. Get wet.

Do your exercises with intensity, for however long you can do them at first, and get to know what it feels like when

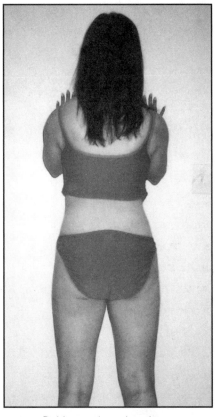

AFTER: Debbie got her adrenaline pumping, and those love handles just had to let go!

your body starts pumping adrenaline. Just like Debbie, you'll want to experience that feeling again and again.

When her fifteenth high school reunion comes around, the only thing Debbie will be spreading is the word that if she can shrink her hot spot, anyone can.

Debbie not only beat the spread, she obliterated it.

A 7-MINUTE SUCCESS

■ STEVE D., 20

A SMOOTH OPERATOR STANDS A CUT ABOVE

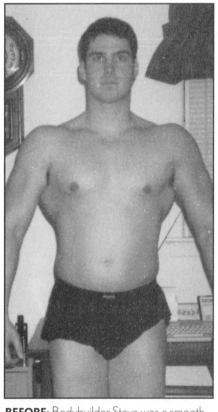

Steve D. is a college student. You can see from his before photo that he had a muscular, powerful physique, but not a refined, defined one. Which is exactly what he would need as he prepared to enter his first bodybuilding contest.

His training goal was to get his abs "cut up," to define his abdominal muscles by losing fat but without losing muscle mass at the same time. Losing muscle mass is a catastrophe for a bodybuilder.

So is being smooth.

In bodybuilding lingo, "smooth" means that the com-

BEFORE: Bodybuilder Steve was a smooth operator, all right—especially around the stomach.

petitor has too much fat covering their muscles. As you can see, Steve was definitely a smooth operator, especially around the stomach.

Smooth is bad, cuts are good. Steve received excellent coaching, working hard to chip the fat away from his abdominal region, making his muscles stand out. Happily, he placed first in his class. There are a few points worth going through.

First, notice how muscular he is at only 20 years old. Steve is living proof that scientists are on the right path by digging into the genetics and not the mechanics of muscle building. Many of you could work out for decades and not achieve one-third of Steve's degree of muscularity.

It doesn't matter what kind of workout you try or how hard you exercise. Weight training can only take you as far as your genes will let you. Keep this in mind the next time some buff TV workout maestro or celebrity tells you that to look like them, all you have to do is exercise and eat like they do.

Since you don't have their genes (unless you're related to them!) and they don't have yours, you might as well face facts: You're never going to look like them. And that's perfectly fine. No matter what your genetic makeup is, learn how to work with your own body. Don't worry so much about theirs!

The rule of thumb when it comes to building muscle is that what you do is not as important as who you are!

Bodybuilders aren't geneticists, but they know what they see. Without the proper body structure ordained at birth and genetic ability to pack on muscle, you cannot become a top-flight competitor. It's as if the top men and women are genetic mutants!

Dr. Paul Thompson, a cardiologist at Hartford Hospital in Connecticut and a muscle-gene connection researcher, put it best: "Some people get big just by walking by the barbells. Others can lift weights a lot and their muscles don't grow much."

The second point is an obvious one. Even with all of his weight training and his tender age, Steve still had a spot fat problem!

The third point is this: No matter what your level of experience, you can do it all by yourself. I told you that Steven received excellent coaching.

He did, but not from me.

Steve goes to school in Pennsylvania and I only get to see him on school breaks.

His trainer was smart enough to use a series of continuous ab exercises in an aerobic manner to burn Steve's fat away. The routine was so tough that Steve only lasted a few minutes each session. He then followed two of the oldest bodybuilder tricks in the book: not eating immediately after working out, and eating a low-fat, moderate-carbohydrate meal.

You probably are smiling at this point, because you realize that Steve was actually following a modified form of the three-step Genetic Body Sculpting method.

Instinctively, he combined specific exercises without weights for a particular body part and worked that area continuously, without counting sets and repetitions. Yet, Steve didn't work out long enough to stimulate his appetite and he took a food pause once he finished exercising.

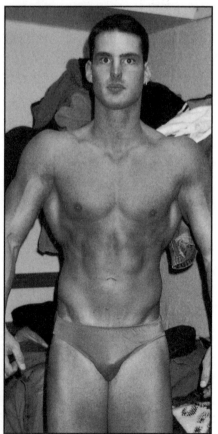

AFTER: Steve contributes yet another "six-pack" to college dorm life!

When he did eat, he followed the blueprint most top contenders swear by. They know that if they are trying hard to lose body fat before a contest, it makes no sense to eat cheeses, fatty meats, or anything fried, which only piles on more fat.

Plus, as you know, it puts your weight control genes to sleep.

Like all bodybuilders, Steve ate more protein than we advocate, but that makes little difference, because as you may recall, dietary protein has little effect on weight-control genes.

As you can see from the after photo, Steve put his weight-control genes to work for him, sculpting his belly fat away.

Congratulations, young man.

A 7-MINUTE SUCCESS

◼ LINDA D., 38

A FAREWELL TO FLABBY ARMS

Which body part do men want to make larger and women smaller?

Give up?

It's the arms, and this difference between the sexes gets played out early. Ask a little boy to show you his muscles and they will immediately hit a double overhead biceps bodybuilding pose.

Ask a little girl to show you her muscles and she'll usually just extend her arm straight out so that *you* can find her muscles.

The size of your arm and the source of your real strength

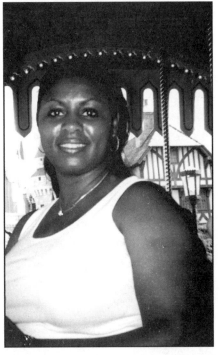

BEFORE: Linda was on a merry-go-round of diets and exercises that did nothing to slim down her "cannon-sized" arms.

come from the three-headed triceps muscle on the back and sides of the upper arm, not the two-headed biceps muscle in the front.

Yet, in our culture, the front of the arm is more highly prized and glamorous than the back. Boys want big biceps, big guns. They want bulging, baseball biceps with the peak of a bishop's miter.

Girls generally couldn't care less.

That is, unless they put on weight as they age, making the back of their arms a soft and fleshy hot spot. That's when it's time for thinner, better defined arms.

Hormones account for much of the differing gender approach to arms. Estrogen, among others, promotes fat storage in the back of the arms, while testosterone promotes muscle tissue build-up in the front part of the arm, explaining why the biceps area usually has little fat.

But that's not always the case.

ARMS CONTROL

I remember a 40-year-old mother of two from New York who had the biggest arms I had ever seen. These were two bulky, bulging cannons. I have 18½-inch arms. Hers were closer to 22 inches.

Incredibly, she had had liposuction done to them 3 years before! Then how did they get so big?

It's hard to believe, but fat from her triceps muscle migrated downward and engulfed her biceps muscle, like green slime. The liposuction apparently did not get rid of enough fat cells and the ones that were left behind filled up to twice their size.

Unlike the other four hot spots, arms have an inherent timing factor that can make slimming them more difficult than the other four hot spots. The longer that fat stays around the triceps, the tougher it is to lose because connective tissue that holds fat cells in bunches gets stretched out, making the arms lax.

Arms are not only a hot spot, they are a tell-tale spot, as well. You can often identify a woman who lost a lot of weight just by looking at her arms because they resist returning to normal size.

The arms may be hard nuts to crack, but if you pay them a bit of extra attention, you can work wonders.

Look what it did for Linda D. from Saddle River, New Jersey.

Linda, an interior designer and mother of a 10-year-old boy, had big guns herself, a posterior arm anomaly that she inherited from her mother and grandmother. Though overweight all over, her arms stood out like a zebra at a lions' convention.

She joined a commercial weight loss center near her house, where she did quite well. However, her arms weren't evaporating fast enough to suit her. So she tried resistance training: weights, rubber cables, and metal springs.

Each did nothing for her arms.

When I first saw her, I explained that resistance training builds muscle, but does not get rid of fat. She needed something that would target her fat, so she began doing The 7-Minute Miracle arms workout along with the post-exercise eating plan.

Within 3 weeks, she lost so much size from her arms that they took over the lead from the rest of her body, spearheading her entire weight-loss effort.

In 90 days, as you can see from the picture below, she turned herself into someone who is armed and dangerous!

AFTER: Linda worked the 7-Minute Miracle arms workout. Now she's proudly "armed and dangerous"!

Linda's story illustrates that any hot spot is fair game, ripe for shrinkage, even if you are very overweight.

You can easily incorporate The 7-Minute Miracle plan into most commercial weight-loss plans, using it to focus on that one tough area just like Linda did.

That's how you, too, can say farewell to flabby arms—forever.

INDEX